**Introductory Biomechanics**

For Elsevier

Commissioning Editor: Rita Demetriou-Swanwick
Development Editor: Natalie Meylan
Project Manager: Vijayakumar Sekar
Designer/Design Direction: Stewart Larking
Illustration Manager: Merlyn Harvey

Introductory Biomechanics

Andy Kerr PhD

Lecturer,
School of Health and Social Care,
Glasgow Caledonian University,
Glasgow, UK

Illustrations by

Antbits

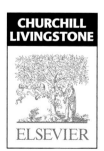

Edinburgh London New York Oxford Philadelphia St Louis Sydney Toronto 2010

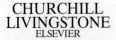

CHURCHILL LIVINGSTONE
ELSEVIER

First published 2010, © Elsevier Limited. All rights reserved.

ISBN 978-0-443-06944-4
  Reprinted 2012 (twice)

British Library Cataloguing in Publication Data
A catalogue record for this book is available from the British Library

Library of Congress Cataloging in Publication Data
A catalog record for this book is available from the Library of Congress

Notice
Knowledge and best practice in this field are constantly changing. As new research and experience broaden our knowledge, changes in practice, treatment and drug therapy may become necessary or appropriate. Readers are advised to check the most current information provided (i) on procedures featured or (ii) by the manufacturer of each product to be administered, to verify the recommended dose or formula, the method and duration of administration, and contraindications. It is the responsibility of the practitioner, relying on their own experience and knowledge of the patient, to make diagnoses, to determine dosages and the best treatment for each individual patient, and to take all appropriate safety precautions. To the fullest extent of the law, neither the Publisher nor the Author assumes any liability for any injury and/or damage to persons or property arising out of or related to any use of the material contained in this book.
  Neither the Publisher nor the Author assumes any responsibility for any loss or injury and/or damage to persons or property arising out of or related to any use of the material contained in this book. It is the responsibility of the treating practitioner, relying on independent expertise and knowledge of the patient, to determine the best treatment and method of application for the patient.

The Publisher

 ELSEVIER your source for books, journals and multimedia in the health sciences
www.elsevierhealth.com

Working together to grow
libraries in developing countries
www.elsevier.com | www.bookaid.org | www.sabre.org
ELSEVIER   BOOK AID International   Sabre Foundation

The Publisher's policy is to use **paper manufactured from sustainable forests**

Printed in China

Table of contents

Acknowledgements

In completing this book over the past 12 months I have relied on the goodwill of several individuals. They are: My father, Andy Kerr, for providing numerous original and creative images as well as some technical advice. My wife, Caroline Kerr, for proof-reading several chapters. The technical team at Glasgow Caledonian University—Danny Rafferty, Gordon Morlan and Gayle Mackie—for valuable advice and practical assistance. Mandy Abbott for the Podiatry images.

In addition I would like to acknowledge my colleagues and former students at Glasgow Caledonian University and University of Nottingham for their feedback and enthusiasm in the development of this material.

Finally I would like to thank Stephen Wilson for his creativity and technical wizardry in developing the interactive DVD without which this project would seem pretty two-dimensional.

Dedication

This book is dedicated to Caroline, Ailsa, Campbell and Flora.

Introduction

This book is intended for students studying a health or sports course that includes some biomechanics. This will include students of physiotherapy, podiatry, occupational therapy, kinesiology, sports therapy and sports science. There are plenty of other textbooks on biomechanics; this book is different because it is specifically aimed at students who have successfully avoided studying physics at any level or still feel nervous about the subject. This also applies to those of you who have forgotten all about biomechanics since you were an undergraduate: you know who you are.

Biomechanics is the study of mechanical force in living bodies. We could call it 'the mechanics of humans' as the bodies in this case are human, although we will be drawing some comparisons with other animals, such as penguins. Understanding how force can produce movement, lead to injury or, when applied by health and sports professionals, aid rehabilitation and enhance sports performance is a central component for many undergraduate and postgraduate courses in health and sport. Biomechanics, like most subjects, can be difficult to grasp but is surprisingly easy if you stick to understanding basic principles which really underpin all the sections of the book, from understanding how muscles move joints to energy conservation during sport.

My experiences in teaching biomechanics to sports science students, physiotherapists and podiatrists has taught me three things: (1) if students had intended to study mechanics they would have applied for engineering; (2) students need material needs to be applied to their area of practice; and (3) students are happier studying material that is interactive and widely illustrated with animations and drawings, especially students interested in human movement. These experiences led to the idea for this book and associated interactive CD-ROM which I hope you will enjoy or at the very least will help you to grasp some of the fundamental principles of biomechanics.

Before we start there are a few things to mention about the design of the book and operation of the CD-ROM.

- You *don't* need any prior knowledge of physics or mathematics but if you do have some knowledge this book will still offer an opportunity to revise your knowledge as well as to apply it to your area of professional practice.

- You *do* need access to a PC or Mac to use the interactive CD-ROM. If you don't have access to one, you can still get a lot from the book but you will miss the parts that really bring the subject to life. You don't need any special software but you will need a CD or DVD drive.

- Each chapter begins with a list of the things you will learn. Take it as a warning of what's to come but also as a way to evaluate your learning; once you have completed the section look back at the 'what you will learn' list—did you get it all? If you think you have then try some of the activities on the CD-ROM.

- The book is based around solving problems which requires some effort on your part. In my experience this is the key to real understanding. Simple recall knowledge might get you through the exams (if you are lucky) but you will fall short when the patient or athlete is in front of you. You may choose not to work out all the details but you should give each question some thought. The answers and explanations to some of the questions are included at the back of the book.

- When you see the CD-ROM symbol 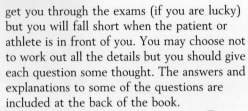 this means there are interactive activities on that topic on your CD-ROM.

- Finally the practical activities are designed to help you understand some of the principles in a practical kind of a way. If you avoid them you may miss out on a key bit of understanding (as well as some fun). If some of the activities are difficult then you can always use your imagination.

Chapter **One**

1

Fundamentals of Force

What you will learn about in this chapter

1. What mechanical force is;
2. What a force does;
3. How you describe a force.

Words you will come across

Force, mass, vector, scalar, Cartesian, magnitude, lever, moment

Force is the very essence of biomechanics, and therefore this book. For this reason the first four chapters will be dedicated entirely to understanding force; what it is, how you describe it, what it does and some principles of analysis. In the first chapter we will focus on some of the basics: what it is, what it does and the conventions of describing a force.

What is force?

It is difficult to encapsulate all that the word 'force' means as it is so elemental to our physical world. It is easier, perhaps, to think of its effect on bodies. (This doesn't necessarily mean the human body. It really means any rigid block of mass. So this could be a steel box, a wooden door or a human femur, anything providing it has mass and keeps its shape.) Simply put: **force changes the motion of bodies**.

There are many different types of force; for example: electromagnetic force, nuclear force and even spiritual force. In this book, we will be talking about **mechanical force**, which you can think of as a **push** or **pull**, e.g. the push on a wheelchair to set it in motion or the pull on a rope during a tug of war.

What does mechanical force do?

Mechanical force is an interaction (or exchange) between bodies that results in a change in motion of all the interacting bodies. This could be a change in the speed of the body, e.g. resting to moving or moving slowly to moving fast, or it could mean a change in the direction of the body. If this sounds a little abstract, too 'sciency', think about the collision between the white ball and a group of coloured balls in a game of pool: the *push* from the white ball at impact causes the coloured balls (as well as the white itself) to move off in all kinds of directions and velocities.

Force can also cause a change in the shape of a body, like a cushion being squashed when you sit on it or a bone being crushed from the impact of a car crash. We will consider this deforming effect of forces in Chapters 6 and 7, but for now let's just think of force as something that changes motion.

Take a simple activity like walking or throwing a ball; behind each change in speed or direction of each part of your body lies a force. Understanding force is clearly important if training (or re-training) movement is one of your objectives. Since this is very relevant to those of you interested in rehabilitation or sport, let's begin this understanding with some important information on force.

Scalar or vector?

To describe any physical **quantity** (length, weight, temperature, speed, etc.) you can just state its magnitude (the **amount** of stuff it has). For example, you might say that a fluid has 200 cubic metres (m^3) of volume or that the wind has a speed of 15 miles per hour, temperature could also be described in terms of a quantity, e.g. 50 degrees Celsius (°C), and I am sure you can think of many others.

If you *only* need magnitude to describe something then the thing you are describing is what we call a **scalar**, such as temperature and volume. To describe a **vector**, on the other hand, we need to know details of the direction of the quantity. Force is a vector since we need to say that it is applied in a particular direction: up, down, east, west. Vector is one of those universal words, used in lots of different situations by different people often to mean different things. Pilots will say they are flying along a specific vector, which is simply the line in the sky they are following, whereas meteorologist might describe a wind vector (you are probably familiar with weather maps and all the little wind arrows (see Fig. 1.1)). To a geneticist a vector is a fragment of DNA used to modify another DNA molecule. In biomechanics the important thing to remember about a vector is that it must have a direction.

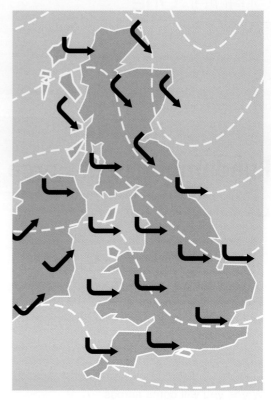

Figure 1.1 • Weather map showing wind vectors.

Practical Activity Box 1.1

In the list below identify the quantities that are scalar and those that are vectors (i.e. need a direction).

Speed	Depth	Circumference	Displacement
Length	Force	Luminosity	Distance
Mass	Heat	Velocity	Acceleration
Wind	Snowfall	Weight	Time

Answer provided in Appendix 1.

Some of these terms seem similar, synonymous even, for example, speed with velocity, distance with displacement. These terms appear to mean the same thing and many people do regard them as the same, which is OK unless you need precision in your language. Distance for example is actually a scalar since you only need to state the amount, e.g. 10 miles or 15 km. Displacement on the other hand is a vector which requires a statement on direction, e.g. 10 miles in a north-westerly direction. An illustration might help.

If you drive from Aberdeen to Birmingham then back to Aberdeen you will have travelled a **distance** of 846 miles or 1364 km, unless of course you live in the USA in which case you will, have travelled 2612 miles (Aberdeen, South Dakota, to Birmingham, Alabama). Regardless of the country, **displacement** will be zero since there has been no change in position, therefore no direction.

It is important that we use the same units to describe a quantity or at least you can accurately convert one system to another; otherwise we would constantly be making errors. In this book, we will be using the International Systems of Units (SI units). Table 1.1 provides some of the typical SI units used in biomechanics and some equivalent units, mainly from the imperial system used, predominantly, in the United Kingdom and USA.

Table 1.1 Quantities used in biomechanics with their SI units and some equivalents

Quantity	Name	SI abbreviation	Equivalent
Base units			
Mass	kilogram	kg	Imperial weights 1 kg = 2.2 lb
Distance	metre	m	Imperial distance 1 m = 3.28 ft
Time	second	s	Nautical time 1 bell = 1,800 s
Temperature	kelvin	K	Celsius 1 K = −272°
Derived values			
Velocity	Metre per second	m/s	Imperial speed 1 m/s = 2.24 miles per hour (mph)
Acceleration	metre per second per second	m/s^2	Gravity $1 m/s^2 = 0.101G$
Area	square metre	m^2	Imperial area $1 m^2 = 10.76 ft^2$
Volume	cubic metre	m^3	Imperial volume $1 m^3 = 220$ gal
Density	kilogram per cubic metre	kg/m^3	Imperial density $1 kg/m^3 = 0.16$ oz/gal
Special units			
Force	newton*	N	Imperial 0.22 pounds of force
Pressure/stress	pascal*	Pa	N/m^2
Energy, work	joule*	J	1 J = 0.24 cal
Angle	radian*	rad	1 rad = 57.3°
Power	watt (J/s)*	W	1 W = 0.0013 horsepower
Derived values from special units			
Moment of force	newton metres	Nm	1 Nm = 0.74 lb ft
Specific energy	joules per kilogram	J/kg	1 J/kg = 0.0024 kcal/kg

*Special units are a historical legacy; typically, the units are named after the individual who first described or measured the quantity, e.g. force being measured in newtons after Sir Isaac Newton (more about him later). These units traditionally are lower-case when spelled out but abbreviated as a capital letter.

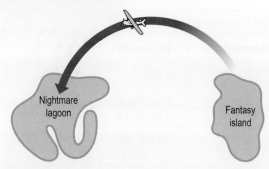

Figure 1.2 • Flight path vector.

Scalar quantities are easy to add or subtract (provided they have the same units) but vectors are a little trickier. But because they have a direction, you can draw them as arrows, which is a bit like flight navigators plotting their vector (flight path (Fig. 1.2)) across the sky or meteorologists drawing wind arrows over maps of different countries.

Drawing vectors

To draw a vector you first need a reference frame. This is just a defined space like the Cartesian graph with X and Y axes that you are probably familiar with from geography and mathematics classes at school. The X axis is the horizontal line with positive values going towards the right and the Y axis is the vertical line with values increasing as you go up (see Fig. 1.3). These axes are perpendicular to each other; i.e. they cross each other at a right angle (90°). In biomechanics this is sometimes referred to

as **orthogonal**, which is simply a fancy way of saying they are at right angles to each other.

This frame defines the space that the force (or any other vector) is acting within. The direction of the axis is defined by the arrowhead at its end. This will tell you whether the vector is positive or negative. For example force **A** (Fig. 1.3) is positive horizontally since it is acting in the same direction as the horizontal (X) axis. If the arrow head was pointing in the opposite direction it would be negative.

The magnitude (amount) of force is represented in a force vector diagram by the length of the arrow, so first you need to decide on an appropriate way to translate the force magnitude value into a length value. A scaling factor if you like. For example, 10 N could equal 1 cm so a force with a magnitude of 35 N would be represented by a line 3.5 cm long. The angle of the force is defined using one of the axes (X or Y) for reference, so it may be 0° to the X axis (which would be the same as 90° to the Y axis) or it could be 30° to the X axis. In Figure 1.3, force **A** has a magnitude of 50 N, so the arrow length (using our scaling factor) is 5 cm. The force is positive along the X axis (arrow pointing in the same direction as X) and is orientated parallel (0°) to the X axis.

Can you translate force **B** (assuming the same scaling factor of 10 N=1 cm)? (Clue: you will need a ruler for magnitude.)

This is easy for straight vectors but what if the force is being applied at an angle, for example **C**? For this you will also need a protractor to measure the angle as well as a ruler. So force **C** has a magnitude of 35 N and is acting down to the right at an angle of 30° to the vertical axis (Y). Can you now do the same for force **D** (40 N)? (Answer is in Appendix 1.)

Some of you may have noticed that we live in three dimensions (four if you consider time, but let's not get carried away). The point is that force also exists in three dimensions, so we need to add in another dimension. If we have X and Y then we must have Z. Like the X axis the Z axis is horizontal (parallel to ground) and 90° to the other two axes. If you have studied anatomy this would be synonymous with the mediolateral direction. If you haven't studied anatomy think of it as side-to-side direction as opposed to forward and back (X) and up and down (Y).

You can use the right-hand rule to understand this relationship: Put your right hand out as if you were going to shake someone's hand (thumb pointing up).

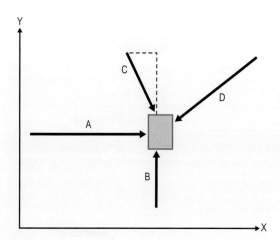

Figure 1.3 • *XY* graph showing forces acting on a box.

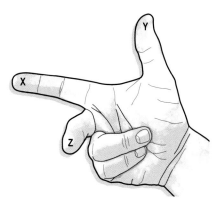

Figure 1.4 • Right-hand rule.

Now close your ring finger and pinkie and point your middle finger to the left. The *Y* is your thumb (positive values in direction thumb is pointing), the *X* your index finger (positive values in direction finger is pointing) and the middle finger is the *Z* axis (positive values in direction finger is pointing); see Figure 1.4. This is the convention used in biomechanics, although some countries use a different combination of *XYZ* to denote the three axes, a typical alternative being *Z* is your thumb (vertical), *Y* is your index (forward and back) and *X* is your middle finger (side to side). If you are still confused then try Activity 1.2.

Practical Activity Box 1.2

Get a piece of blank paper and mark two axes, *X* and *Y*. Now get your pencil (sharpened) and push it through the point where they cross (the origin). You now have the three axes, *X*, *Y* on the paper and your pencil is *Z*.

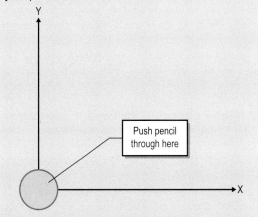

Figure 1.5 • Illustration of paper for practical activity 1.2.

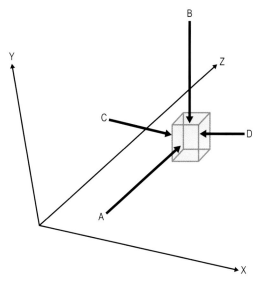

Figure 1.6 • *XYZ* graph showing forces acting on a box.

The important thing is to avoid confusion by knowing which convention the textbook, scientific journal or movement laboratory is using. In this textbook we will be using the one shown in Figure 1.4.

As we have said forces acting in the same direction as the axes will have a positive value; however, forces acting in the opposite direction will have negative values but this doesn't mean the push or pull of force is less than 0. It is simply acting in the opposite direction.

Force **B** in Figure 1.6 is a vertical force of −60 N since it is acting in the opposite direction to the *Y* axis, i.e. downwards. Force **A** has a magnitude of 50 N in the *Z* direction.

Point of application

From what we have talked about so far we know that force has magnitude (length of arrow), direction (arrowhead) and angle (in relation to axes), all defined within our *XYZ* reference frame. But does it matter where the force is actually applied (i.e. the tip of the arrow) on the object, e.g. on the box or bone?

Put your pen or pencil on the table in front of you. Now you are going to:

1. Apply a pushing force, more or less at the centre of the pencil.

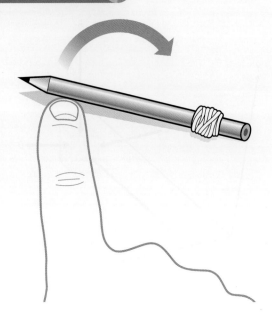

Figure 1.7 • Pencil being pushed.

2. Apply a pushing force (same magnitude as before) at one end of the pencil (see Fig. 1.7).

The movement of the pencil is entirely different, depending on where you applied the force. When the force was applied at the middle of the pencil the whole pencil moved in the direction of the push; however, when the force was applied away from the centre the pencil rotated. The first force caused a linear motion (straight line); the second force caused an angular motion (rotation). A force that causes rotation is called a moment or torque, from the Latin *torquere*, which means to twist. The point where the force is applied is clearly important to the resulting motion and needs to be stated. This is called the **point of application** and is usually expressed by using a reference frame for the object being pushed, i.e. the *X,Y,Z* coordinates of the box, ball or banana.

Force magnitude and change in motion

As we now know **magnitude** is the quantity, or amount, of push or pull represented by the length of the vector in a vector diagram. When we talk about movement, force magnitude is defined from the **acceleration** that the force produces on a

body. Now acceleration needs some clear definition because it doesn't just mean how fast you are moving. Let's start with velocity (which is how fast you are moving):

Velocity = change in displacement divided by time or

$$V = \frac{Position^2 - Position^1}{Time}$$

So if a ball was rolling down a school corridor from position[1] (let's say 3 m along the corridor) to position[2] (let's say 7 m along the corridor) and this took 3 seconds, then the ball had a velocity of

(7 m – 3 m)/3 s = 1.33 metres per second (m/s)

Now acceleration is the rate of change of velocity (or the time derivative of velocity), i.e. how quickly or slowly the velocity of the body is changing, speeding up or slowing down. If velocity is constant then there is no acceleration. The greater the change in velocity the greater the acceleration; this relationship is formalized in the equation for average acceleration:

Acceleration = change in velocity (velocity at end – velocity at start)/time

or

$$A = \frac{Velocity^2 - Velocity^1}{Time}$$

Let's imagine you went up to the ball which was still happily rolling down the corridor and gave it another push (in the same direction that it is was rolling). Before you pushed it the ball had a velocity of 1.33 m/s and after the push (which lasted 2 s) it had a velocity of 2.45 m/s. This would mean there was an acceleration of

2.45 m/s – 1.33 m/s divided by 2 = 0.56 metres per second per second (m/s/s)

During your push, the ball increased its velocity by 0.56 m/s every second.

Acceleration is a vector, like force, and can be described as positive (velocity increasing, i.e. getting faster) or negative (velocity decreasing, i.e. getting slower), which is also known as deceleration. In

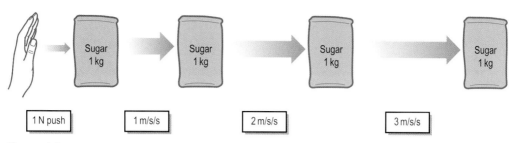

Figure 1.8 • Acceleration of a 1-kg object from an application of a 1 N force (push).

his ground-breaking book *Principia Mathematica* (1687) Sir Isaac Newton laid down the rules which govern how force causes motion. In recognition of this achievement force magnitude is measured in newtons, where 1 newton (N) is the amount of force required to accelerate a 1 kg of mass by 1 m/s every second. We will talk abut these laws in more detail in Chapter 4; however, it is worth remembering that force causes acceleration, or a change in velocity.

If you imagine a 1 kg bag of sugar and apply 1 N to it then the bag would move (provided we ignore all other forces such as friction and air resistance) in the direction the force is applied, getting faster by 1 m/s, every second for the duration of the push (see Fig. 1.8).

Let's add a bit of modern technology to Newton's well-known analogy of the falling apple to understand the force of gravity. If you knew that an apple was about to fall from a tree and managed to set up a high-speed camera to record the fall the developed photographs would show the apple falling a greater and greater distance between each photograph; i.e. the velocity of the apple (distance divided by time) was increasing. If, on the other hand, you lived in space with zero gravity (although admittedly it would be a little strange to find a productive apple tree in space) and photographed the same falling apple, there would be the same distance between each snapshot of the apple; i.e. it would be moving at the same velocity throughout its fall. Of course in the absence of gravity we would need some force to actually start the apple moving in the first place! We will talk more later about falling objects.

Of course, acceleration is not just about gravity; *every* force causes a body to accelerate. We will return to acceleration and Sir Isaac Newton in later chapters but for now let's recap on what we know about force.

What you need to remember so far

A mechanical force is basically a **push** or a **pull** that causes a body to **accelerate**. To describe a force accurately you need to remember that it is a **vector** with four characteristics:

1. **Magnitude**, which is measured in newtons (N);
2. **Direction**, which is defined using a standard reference frame like the *XYZ* Cartesian frame in Figure 1.6;
3. **Point of application** on the body, again using standard reference frame; and
4. **Angle of application**, in degrees or radians.

The force of muscles

Within the human body force is produced through the contraction of skeletal muscle. This could mean the muscles shortening (known as a concentric contraction), lengthening while tense (known as an eccentric contraction) or being in a state of tension while remaining at the same length (known as a static or isometric contraction). These types of contraction are demonstrated in Figure 1.9 with the quadriceps muscle group. In the first diagram the knee is straightening, produced by **shortening** of the quadriceps. In the second diagram the knee is flexing; this movement is produced by gravity, although the movement is still controlled by the quadriceps, the muscle lengthening while producing tension. In the final diagram the knee is being held in the same position; gravity is still trying to pull the leg down but the quadriceps are matching this force with a static contraction—no movement.

◉ CD-ROM activity 1.1: video

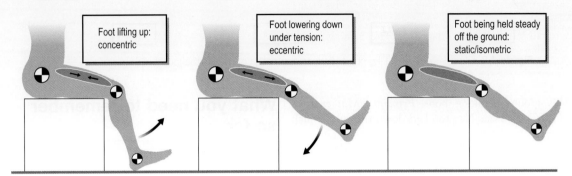

Figure 1.9 • Types of muscle contraction.

It is worth noting that although we can apply pushing **and** pulling forces on an object, our muscles always **pull** on bones, never push, which makes things a little easier to understand. Also, muscles are not intelligent: they behave very simply, and can produce only one type of contraction at a time—isometric, concentric or eccentric.

The direction and angle of the muscle **pull** are defined by the anatomy of the muscle, in particular the location of the tendinous attachments on the bone (point of application). The magnitude of the pull corresponds, in general, to the size of the muscle, that is, its physiological cross-sectional area, or how thick it is. However, it is the brain (motor cortex to be exact) that determines how many muscle fibres are active at any one point, a bit like the conductor in an orchestra pointing to just a couple of cellos when a gentle soft sound is required, or the whole ensemble for a crescendo.

An important mechanical feature of the force generated by most skeletal muscles is that it is applied at a distance from the centre of a joint (Fig. 1.10), like when you pushed the pencil at the end rather than at the centre. This is particularly true of muscles in the body that create motion; these are sometimes referred to as mobilizer muscles.

The importance of this distance between where the force is applied and the joint or fulcrum is best illustrated with a simple experiment.

Walk over to a door and pull it open. Where did you apply your pulling force?

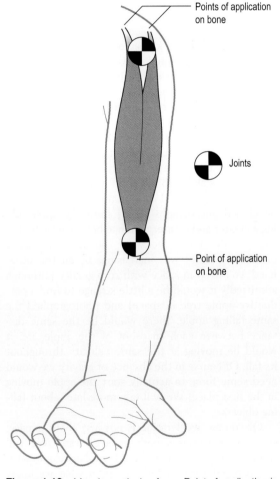

Points of application on bone

Joints

Point of application on bone

Figure 1.10 • Muscle producing force. Point of application is beyond the joint centre.

I like to think you all did the same thing there (the handle is a bit of a clue!). The point is, like the mobilizer muscles in your body, you applied your pulling force well away from the joint or in the door's case, the hinges. This is the principle of **moments** and is the basis for the simplest (and most efficient) machine known to man: the **lever**, which we will talk about in Chapter 5. The turning force (moment or sometimes called torque) is created when a force is applied at a distance away from the turning part (this can be called the pivot, fulcrum, hinge or joint). You know the principle of moments intuitively; otherwise, you would sit in the middle of a seesaw!

Of course you know what happens if you sit in the middle of a seesaw so you can work out what happens if you apply a force at the hinges of a door or if a muscle applies its pull at a joint centre. Some muscles are indeed attached so that their pull is close to the joint centre. What function will these muscles perform? They won't rotate the bone, so what do they do? What does your force do when you sit in the middle of the seesaw? Can this force serve any purpose?

In fact these muscles are critical to movement. They fix (or stabilize if you prefer) a body part to enable motion to occur—a bit like the screws in the door hinge holding the bracket in place or the bolt that secures the seesaw to the ground. These muscles are sometimes called stabilizer muscles, for obvious reasons.

Human movement is generally performed through a series of rotations at joints. Think of the number of body parts that turn when you walk: ankle, knee, hip, pelvis, shoulder, elbow. Each rotation is generated and controlled by muscles. To allow these rotations to occur the central axis of the body needs to remain stable. A seesaw that moved about on the ground would prove an awkward toy to play with; it has to be fixed to the ground to allow the rotation to occur. Likewise the muscles attached very close to, or right at, the joint centre act to hold or stabilize the bone.

Magnitude of moments

Like the force that causes linear (straight) motion (for example, the push on a car), moments are also vectors, so we need all the same information as

before. Firstly the magnitude: this is the product (multiplication) of the applied force and its perpendicular (at 90°; see Fig. 1.11) distance from the fulcrum (this distance is also known as the moment or lever arm):

Moment = force (N) × perpendicular distance (m) from pivot

So moments are measured in newton metres (Nm) or equivalents, such as pound feet.

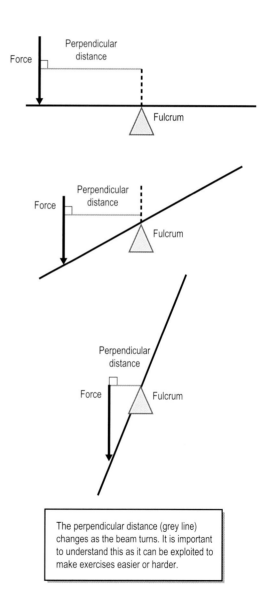

The perpendicular distance (grey line) changes as the beam turns. It is important to understand this as it can be exploited to make exercises easier or harder.

Figure 1.11 • Perpendicular distance.

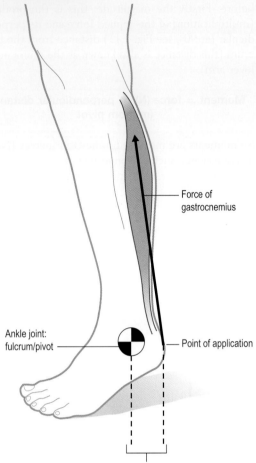

Force of gastrocnemius

Ankle joint: fulcrum/pivot

Point of application

Distance between muscle force application and fulcrum (approx. 0.05 m). Also known as the moment arm.

Figure 1.12 • Plantar flexing (up onto toes) moment created by gastrocnemius (calf muscle) contraction.

Let's say the gastrocnemius muscle (calf) (see Fig. 1.12) pulls on the heel with a force of 150 N and this is applied 5 cm (0.05 m) perpendicularly behind the ankle joint. The turning force is therefore 150 N × 0.05 m = 7.5 Nm. If you had a larger calcaneum (heel bone), say one that extended 8 cm (0.08 m) back from the ankle joint then the turning force will be 12 Nm (150 × 0.08), nearly 40% more for just 3 cm! The point here is that you can change the size of the turning force by changing the distance to the joint, although admittedly changing the size of your calcaneum is a little tricky.

CD-ROM activity 1.2

Let's imagine you were testing the strength of someone's quadricep muscle group (muscles on front of the thigh that straighten the leg) and you ask the person who is sitting on a plinth to straighten their knee while you push against them. Where do you place your hand, i.e. your resisting force?

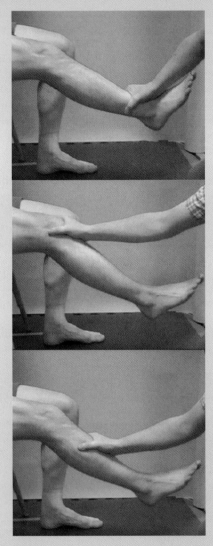

Figure 1.13 • Hand placement to resist knee extension.

Of course you place it furthest away from the joint, giving yourself the longest possible moment arm (perpendicular distance between axis of rotation and point where force is applied). Your force is at a mechanical advantage compared to the poor old quadriceps which applies its pull very close to the knee joint.

Direction of moments

So the magnitude of a moment is force × distance (Nm). Moments are of course vectors so we need to state a direction. As rotation is the resulting motion the convention is to state the moment as positive when it creates a clockwise motion and negative when it creates an anti-clockwise movement. When applied to the body moments can be described in terms of the motion they create about the joint, e.g. a knee flexor moment or a hip abducting moment. The point of application is the same as previously, i.e. the point on the bone (or other object).

 CD-ROM activity 1.3

What you have to remember about moments

Moments are turning forces created by a force applied at a distance from a turning point. The magnitude is the product of force and perpendicular distance from joint. Moments are described as clockwise or anti-clockwise or if applied to the body according to the motion they will produce, for example flexion/extension, adduction/abduction. Forces applied around the centre of a joint help to stabilize it; they do not produce turning motions.

2

Gravity, Mass and Stability

What you will learn about in this chapter

1. The difference between gravity and mass;
2. The centre of mass and how it alters during different postures and movements;
3. A body's stability defined by the base of support and centre of mass;
4. Strategies for remaining balanced; and
5. How gravity creates moments.

Words you will come across

Gravity, mass, centre of mass, gravitational moments, base of support and stability

Gravity: the ultimate force

The force we have to contend with constantly, and one which has literally shaped our bodies, is **gravity**. Gravity is a pulling force. Every piece of mass in the universe pulls other pieces of mass to it. Before you ask why you are not all sticking together, the strength of the pull depends on the amount of the mass; generally you have to have the same mass as a planet before you create a gravitational (pulling) field worth talking about.

Distance is also a factor in the pull of gravity; after all, if gravity was just dependent on mass then all of us would be pulled towards the object with the most mass, e.g. the sun, but the sun is too far away to exert that much of a pull on us individually. Gravity becomes stronger the closer you get to the large mass and weaker the further you are away

from it. Newton (who else!) worked this out and called it the Law of Universal Gravitation. Being a mathematician he expressed this law with a formula:

$$\text{Gravity} = \frac{G \times (\text{mass}^1 \times \text{mass}^2)}{\text{Distance between the two masses squared}}$$

N.B. G is a constant value consistent throughout the universe; the inclusion of this value helps make the equation work (probably best to leave it at that).

The large mass closest to us is, of course, our beloved planet, Earth. The mass of the Earth is constantly pulling us towards its centre. The amount it pulls is measured in terms of how much acceleration (see Chapter 1, Fig. 1.8, for a reminder of acceleration) it produces on bodies located on its surface. This has been measured at 9.81 m/s/s, so every piece of mass on the surface of Earth (and even the air in the atmosphere) is pulled towards its centre at a rate of 9.81 m/s every second. Put it another way, when an object falls to the ground it increases its speed of descent by 22 mph every second(!): 22, 44, 66, etc. It wouldn't take long before it's moving pretty fast. Something to think about before you lean over the side of the Eiffel Tower. We will cover the relationship between force and acceleration in more detail in Chapter 4.

The reason that gravity isn't causing you to move while you are sitting there reading this book (it hasn't just given up or been switched off) is that you have hit a hard block, the ground or any supporting surface. If you didn't have this hard block under you, e.g. if you found yourself falling from a bridge or just after you cleared the bar during a pole vault jump, then you would accelerate downwards. As Galileo demonstrated in 1604 every object accelerates at the same rate on Earth regardless of its weight (see Further Information 2.1). Try it: get a coin and a pen and drop them at the same time (Fig. 2.1).

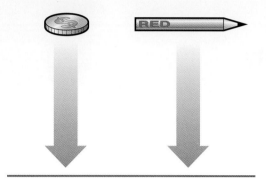

Figure 2.1 • Pen and coin dropped together.

They should have reached the ground at the same time. They didn't!

If you dropped them from a small height, you may not have been quick enough to notice much. If you dropped them from a higher point, you may be ready to argue with me that they don't hit the ground at the same time. They do experience exactly the same accelerating force (gravity); however, the forces that slow them down (decelerating forces) are different. This relates to the shape and smoothness of each falling body (we will talk more about this in Chapter 8), but basically the pen will experience more air resistance than the coin due to its larger surface area in contact with the passing air. Because of this it will slow down more than the coin. If you did the same experiment on the Moon (where there is no air to slow things down) then the objects will definitely hit the ground at the same time, although they will fall slower than on Earth due to the reduced gravity!

Further Information Box 2.1

As an experimental scientist, Galileo Galilei was a bit of a rarity in the seventeenth century; most scientists of the day preferred thought experiments (useful in some ways but lacks the word **evidence** that we are so enamored with in the twenty-first century). Even at the beginning of his career he was unhappy with the untested, yet widely held idea that objects of different weight fell at different speeds. I would guess that some people today still believe it to be true, and to be honest it doesn't seem so weird under casual observation. But Galileo was not one for casual observation; he wanted to test it and in Italy there are some handy leaning towers to help inquisitive scientists. From the leaning tower of Pisa (yes, it was leaning even then) Galileo dropped objects of various mass (but of similar size and shape) at the same time: cannon balls, wooden balls, musket balls and balls made of different metals. When he found that the objects, (more or less) hit the ground at the same time the accepted wisdom (championed by Aristotle; more on him later) was rejected and Galileo's hypothesis, that every object is subjected to the same acceleration (gravity), was accepted. This is also know as the equivalence principle and was the foundation for Newton's Laws of Motion (Chapter 4). The falling objects are subjected to different amounts of friction and air resistance (depending on their shape) which explains why we perceive heavier objects to fall to the ground faster than lights ones.

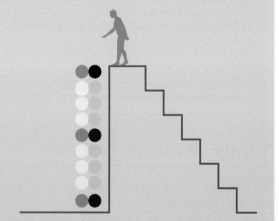

Figure 2.2 • Dropping objects of different size from a leaning tower.

In fact astronaut David Scott repeated Galileo's experiment on the Moon using a falcon feather and a hammer (it could have been anything really) and found that without air resistance they did indeed fall at the same rate.

Historians still debate whether Galileo actually conducted the experiment, but whether he did or didn't, he was right, as thousands of schoolchildren and the odd astronaut can testify to.

Because the Moon is smaller than the Earth (around a sixth of the mass) it has less gravity (around a sixth that of Earth's). This means that visitors to the Moon like Buzz Aldrin and Neil Armstrong felt less of a downward pull when they were walking about on the Moon's surface, illustrating the difference between weight and mass. Let me explain: the astronauts had more or less the same amount of mass as they had when on Earth and yet if they stood on a weighing scale on the Moon they would weigh less (around a sixth) than they did on Earth because there is less of a force pulling them down (gravity). So weight is the amount of mass you have multiplied by the acceleration of gravity (which may vary according to the planet you are living on).

Put another way, weight will vary according to the accelerations the body is experiencing, whereas mass is simply the amount of stuff you have contained within the confines of your skin which won't alter (well not easily or quickly). Although both are confusingly measured in kilograms, weight is really synonymous with force. We will talk a bit more about this later but if you didn't understand that why not try Practical Activity 2.1.

Practical Activity Box 2.1

This is quite a fun experiment that will demonstrate the difference between mass and weight as well as showing you a really easy and quick way to lose weight. Get a set of analogue weighing scales (ones with a dial not digital) and go to one of the lifts in your building (if you don't have access to a lift, don't worry; there are alternatives mentioned at the end). Now, making sure you have the lift to yourself, stand on the scales and take a note of your weight. Now press the up button while looking at your dial. What happened? Did your weight momentarily increase? Next time I want you to press the down button and watch the dial again. This time your weight should drop; although brief, it isn't a long-term alternative to dieting if you want to lose weight.

So why did you lose and gain weight simply from going up and down in a lift? Let's analyse the forces. First when the lift was standing still (A): You are applying a force (mass × gravity) down onto the weighing scale and it is pushing you back (otherwise you would fall), by exactly the same amount. This push up is what is displayed by the dial. Basically the forces are in balance.

When you pressed the up button, the bottom (B) of the floor started to push up more on your feet (you might even be able to feel your knees buckle a little). This upward acceleration increases your weight. When you pressed down (C), the opposite occurred: the increased downward acceleration means you (temporarily) weigh less. You will notice that these changes are brief and that the scales quickly return to normal, even when you are still moving at a constant velocity. This is because, although you might still be moving, there are no accelerations.

The point to remember here is that a **change** in acceleration alters your weight. You can get the same feeling from a rollercoaster, or even driving over hilly country lanes. Even if you bounce up and down on a set of weighing scales your apparent weight changes, even if your actual weight (mass) remains the same, because you are accelerating.

See CD-ROM activity 2.1 for a look at some weighing scales

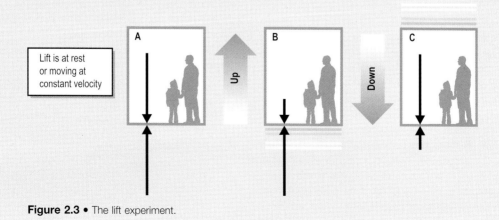

Figure 2.3 • The lift experiment.

The advantages of the Moon's atmosphere; low gravity and lack of air resistance (remember the feather and hammer being dropped) are behind proposals to build a moon base for launching space flights to Mars. In this way the energy cost of lifting a large mass (the shuttle, at lift off, has a total mass of around 109,000 kg) off the surface is much reduced. Also when it comes to landing, the lack of air will not cause the same high temperature that spacecraft experience on re-entry to Earth's atmosphere (the surface of the shuttle can rise to 816°C!) because there is less friction on the vessel's surface from the air.

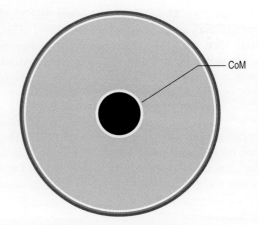

Figure 2.4 ● Centre of mass of a ball filled evenly with foam.

Looks like I have wandered off on a tangent. Let's come back down to Earth and try to understand more about mass, because, as I hope you will see, it is critical to understanding human movement as well as space travel.

Centre of mass

When gravity (or indeed any force) acts on an object, such as your body, it acts on every particle of mass within that body. This makes analysis very difficult, so to simplify this situation (always desirable) we can think of the force acting about a single average point—the centre of mass (CoM).

The CoM is the average position of all the bits of the body's mass. Consequently it will depend on the density (the thickness of the mass) and its distribution within the shape of the body. The CoM of a ball filled with foam would be at its geometric centre (see Fig. 2.4), provided that the ball is a perfect circle of course and the mass (foam) within it is evenly distributed. If the mass was denser (more packed in) at the top than the bottom then the CoM would be higher. The CoM simply reflects where the mass is.

Look around at some of the objects in the room you are in just now—chair, filing cabinet, TV, computer, bookcase, etc.—and try to guess where the CoM is for each one. Don't just pick the centre of the shape; perhaps there are some bits heavier than others, the top of the table for example. There may be empty spaces within the object, e.g. within a personal computer, which can alter the CoM position. Maybe there are some components that are very dense like the screen of a visual display unit.

Calculating the centre of mass

Rather than guess the location of the CoM it may be necessary to calculate its exact position. This is critical for engineers designing large structures such as bridges and office blocks and, although arguably less critical, provides a better understanding of movement and injury in sport and rehabilitation. Various methods for calculating the centre of mass of the human body have been used. In the seventeenth century, the Italian scientist Borelli used balance boards to estimate the CoM location; this worked because the point about which the body balances is the same as the CoM.

Remember those long boring days at school when, instead of listening to your maths teacher, you were busy trying to balance your pencil on your rubber (I'm pretty sure I wasn't the only one (see Fig. 2.5)); well, you were actually doing the same thing as Borelli, finding the pencil's CoM. The balance point on your pencil is the same as its centre of mass. If there were more pencil mass on one side of the rubber than the other then it would tip in the direction of most mass. There must be equal amounts of mass on either side of the pencil for it to be balanced, so the rubber must lie at the CoM.

CD-ROM activity 2.2 Lying on back experiment

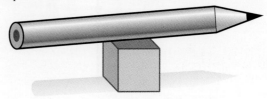

Figure 2.5 ● Balancing a pencil on a rubber.

Practical Activity Box 2.2

To do this activity you will need a wobble board and a strong plank of wood, but if you don't have these things you can just imagine the activity and try CD-ROM activity 2.2 which has a mock-up.

Finding the balance point of a human can be done just at crudely as you balancing the pencil on top of the rubber by using a wobble board. Do not be confused with the instrument used by Rolf Harris to replicate the sound of thunder. By wobble board I mean the mini-seesaw used to train balance. Get a plank of wood and place it on top of the wobble board so that it is balanced. This will need a bit of adjustment. Now get a piece of chalk or similar and draw a line from the point on the ground that the fulcrum touches and then up and over the board (black vertical in Fig. 2.6). Now carefully sit down in the middle of the wobble board (more or less on your chalk line) and slowly lie down. One of three things will happen: either your head end falls down, your feet end falls down or you are balanced. To become balanced will require a little bit of shuffling up or down. Now, when you are finally balanced look at the position of the chalk mark (you may need a friend to help); it should now be at your centre of mass. There is just as much of your mass below the chalk line as above it.

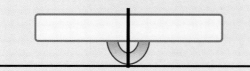

Figure 2.6 • Wobble board for practical activity 2.2.

From this balanced point try lifting your hands up. What should happen and what did happen? Can you explain any movement that occurred? Try moving other parts of your body but before you do, try to predict what might happen.

Of course we have only really estimated the **height** of your CoM. To get a truly three-dimensional location you will need to repeat the experiment in standing. I will let you get on with that in your own time. Estimating the height is good enough for me.

By applying this type of analysis (balancing bodies) to elderly male cadavers research studies have shown that the overall CoM of the human body, when standing upright with arms by the side, lies within the pelvis. To be more precise, it has been

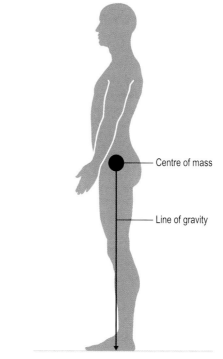

Figure 2.7 • Centre of mass of a typical human in quiet standing: 5 cm in front of the second sacral tuberosity.

placed at 5 cm anterior to the second sacral tuberosity (see Fig. 2.7), the bone at the base of your spine. Sports textbooks sometimes use a value of 55% of height (feet up), which is approximately the same point. (Why not measure it on yourself and see if it is the same?)

I have drawn a line vertically down from the CoM in Figure 2.7. This is the **line of gravity** and is a useful way of understanding posture and movement used by rehabilitation workers and sports professionals. It represents the direction of gravity which is acting through (on average) the CoM.

This may or may not be obvious to you but the CoM does not necessarily have to lie within the mass of the body. The CoM of a doughnut for example is in the centre, i.e. in the hole in the middle. It's just something to bear in mind when you come to analysing body positions.

We have looked at the CoM for quiet (very quiet in the case of the male cadavers) standing; however, we are constantly on the move, changing postures from sitting to lying, standing to walking, standing to swimming, etc. As the CoM represents the location of all the body parts it will change as the body changes. So for example if you move your hands forward, there will be more mass forward than previously so the overall CoM will have moved forward. As soon as you stand up your CoM will also rise, because more of your mass is higher up. On the following group of pictures (Fig. 2.8) put your finger where you think the CoM is located. Think where it was in quiet standing (within pelvis) then look at how the body parts are arranged now. Is there more mass further forwards or further back than in standing, or is it lower or higher.

Hopefully you found that a useful exercise and one that you can practice on real people performing

sport as well as everyday activities. Just be careful not to stare for too long: some people won't understand.

Now of course things are not as simple as looking at a picture or even videos. We have made a big assumption (assumptions are pretty commonplace in biomechanics; otherwise you would keep getting stuck) that mass is evenly distributed within a shape. That there is the same amount of mass within the same area in the legs compared to the trunk is clearly wrong.

Humans are made of different kinds of material, which we will talk about later in Chapter 7, with

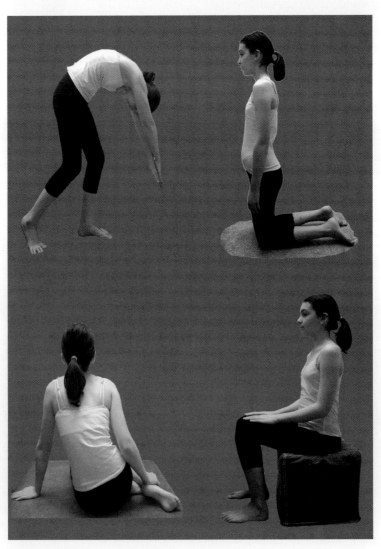

Figure 2.8 • Find the centre of mass.

different amounts of stuff within them. Muscle is one of the most densely packed structures in our bodies and our legs (generally) have the greatest amount of muscle tissue (because of their constant battle against gravity), so basically there is more mass in our legs than in our trunk, which may look large but contains a lot of space (think of the air in your lungs and other organs to a lesser extent). So if we move a leg forward then the CoM will move more than if we had moved our arms or bellies by a similar amount.

What should you remember about mass?

Mass is the amount of stuff within a shape. It is measured in kilograms (kg). It is different from weight which is synonymous with your body force. To make life easier you can represent the whole mass of a body by its CoM. The CoM moves with the body so that it can be outwith the body shape in some circumstances. We will talk more about mass and how it relates to movement in Chapter 4 when we look at Newton's Laws of Motion.

Moments created by mass

Gravity pulls us straight down. I know that's obvious and I have probably laboured the point already, but it's worth remembering. Now that I have got that off my chest we can proceed. Our bodies are made up of lots of linked segments, each with its own mass and therefore a point we can call the segmental CoM (as opposed to the overall CoM we have been talking about previously). Now because each segment is linked by a rotational point (joints) this will mean that gravity (which, on average, will be applied at the segmental CoM) can create moments, which are (if you recall, if not go back to Chapter 1) rotational forces caused by a force being applied about a pivot/hinge/joint. To illustrate this effect of gravity let's try a simple exercise, Practical Activity 2.3.

Moments created by gravity are a useful way of structuring resistance exercises if you were trying to train a group of muscles. Consider the following problem.

An athlete is recovering from a serious shoulder injury. Following a long period in a sling his muscles are very weak generally. You decide to work first on

---

Stand up and move your right arm out to the side (abduction), like you would if you were signaling to turn right on a bike (see Fig. 2.9). Hold it there. You should feel the muscles around your shoulder working pretty hard to hold this abducted position. So, what are your muscles working against? Let's analyse the forces at work:

There is a moment caused by gravity acting directly down (I said you would need to remember that) on the mass of your arm. Now, although gravity is acting on every particle of mass in your arm it can be averaged out to act at the CoM, which is probably around your elbow (depending on how muscular you are), which if I am not mistaken is some distance from your shoulder.

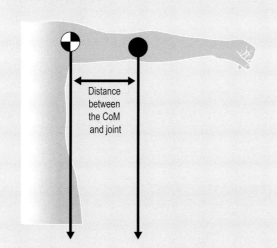

Distance between the CoM and joint

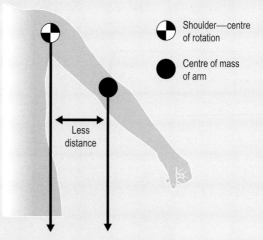

◑ Shoulder—centre of rotation

● Centre of mass of arm

Less distance

Figure 2.9 ● Hold your arm out to the side.

Continued

Practical Activity Box 2.3—cont'd

The force of gravity acting at the CoM of the arm (represented by the line of gravity) will therefore cause an adducting moment about your shoulder; i.e. it is trying to bring your arm down to your side. The size of this moment depends on the mass of your arm (and anything it is holding, weight or cup of coffee) and where this is centred (i.e. CoM) in relation to the joint centre (see Fig. 2.9). So for example if you were wearing a plaster of paris cast on your wrist the CoM would move further down your arm, increasing the distanced from the fulcrum (shoulder), as well as increasing the amount of mass and therefore increasing the adducting moment.

Now bring your arm closer to your body (let's say halfway down) and hold it there. Now, does that feel better?

You should have found that holding your arm closer to your body was easier. The reason for this is the

reduced distance (moment arm) between the line of gravity and centre of rotation. This doesn't mean that your arm has shortened but it has moved through an arc that brings the CoM and centre of rotation closer, reducing the moment. If you continue to move your arm down the CoM will lie more or less directly underneath the centre of rotation. Therefore no moments will be created. Which is why it is easier to walk with your arms by your side than holding them out to the side (just in case you were wondering).

What about if you held your arm out to the side with your elbow bent, how does that change the difficulty? Clue: the CoM of the arm will have moved.

CD-ROM activity 2.3: Your CD-ROM contains another example of this.

strengthening his shoulder abductors (muscles that lift your arm out to the side) by getting him to hold a certain position for 5 s at a time. Which position would be the easiest:

1. Lying on his side with the weak arm raised toward the ceiling at 90°?

2. Standing up with arm raised out to side (i.e. the same position as in Fig. 2.10 but in standing)?

After a couple of sessions he has improved and you would like to introduce more resistance to the

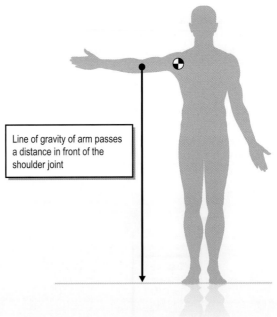

Line of gravity of arm passes a distance in front of the shoulder joint

Figure 2.11 • Position B; Standing up with arm raised out to side (i.e. the same position as A but in standing)?

muscles. How could you alter the position in Fig. 2.11 to create a little bit more resistance to the shoulder abductors? (Answers are in Appendix 2.)

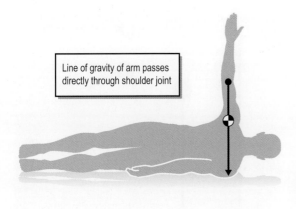

Line of gravity of arm passes directly through shoulder joint

Figure 2.10 • Position A; Lying on side with the weak arm raised toward the ceiling at 90°?

Let's try another one: following a hip replacement operation the hip abductor muscles (muscles that move the leg out to the side; predominantly this is gluteus medius) are generally weak due to the damage from the surgery on the lateral side of the hip. You are not sure which exercises to start with so you decide on the easiest ones for the hip abductors. Considering the moments caused by gravity (don't forget: it pulls things directly down!) place the following positions in order of difficulty, with the most difficult first:

a) The patient lying on their back moving the operated leg out into abduction (out to side).

b) Standing and moving operated leg out into abduction.

c) Lying on 'good' side and lifting operated leg directly up into abduction.

d) Lying on 'good' side with knee bent and moving leg directly up into abduction.

See Appendix 2 for answer.

This simple exercise illustrates the moments created by gravity and has hopefully presented you with some logical ideas for making an exercise easier or indeed more difficult.

Moments and posture

Of course, moments created by gravity are not limited to when we move one of our limbs. Think about your sitting position at the moment and in particular your head. If, like in Fig. 2.12, your head is jutting forward on your neck (if it isn't, then just try it for a few moments) then the CoM of the head will be placed relatively forward on the neck. What does this mean for muscle effort?

The downward force, created by gravity acting on the mass of the head, will be located at the CoM. Poking your head forward moves this CoM (and therefore the force) forward from the joints in the neck, thereby creating a turning force which is trying to flex the neck (bring the head down onto the chest). If this is difficult to imagine then try to think what would happen if someone came up to you and pushed down on your head, with it still poking forward; in this position it would flex down. This is exactly what gravity is trying to do.

So why doesn't your head fall down? And why will this posture lead to discomfort and how could you relieve this discomfort (without resorting to painkillers)? (Answers are in Appendix 2.)

Considering gravitational moments and stability of segments what would the ideal posture look like? Don't think about aesthetics but rather a posture that creates the least amount of muscle work and causes the least amount of stress on tissues.

From what we have previously said about gravitational moments the ideal standing posture would be one that places the CoM of each segment close to the joint centre, like a stack of children's play blocks all squarely placed on top of each other. This minimizes any turning force in the same way that sitting in the middle of a seesaw means you don't tilt one of the sides down. This will minimize consequent muscle activity. An ideal standing posture has therefore been suggested to be one where the line of gravity, from the head down, passes:

1. Through the mastoid process (the bony lump behind the ear);

2. Just in front of the shoulder joint;

3. Just behind the hip joint;

4. Through or just in front of the knee joint; and

5. A couple of centimetres in front of the ankle joint.

See Figure 2.13.

Stability

Generally what we mean by stability of a rigid body is its ability to return to its original position after experiencing an external force(s), like a push. If a body was unstable its position is likely to change when it is pushed. This could result in a fall and injury or for a sportsman it could mean being

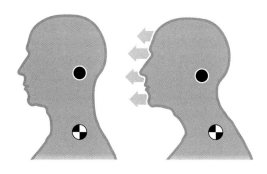

● Centre of mass of head

◓ Centre of rotation in neck

Figure 2.12 • Centre of mass location with good and bad (chin poking forward) neck postures.

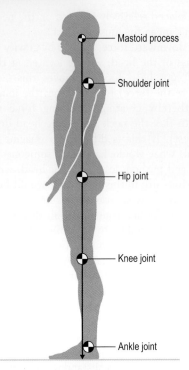

Figure 2.13 • Ideal standing posture.

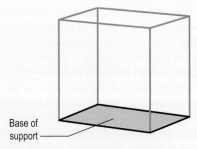

Figure 2.14 • Base of support of a box.

(BoS). This is the area of contact a body has with its supporting surface. For example, a box sitting on the ground has a typically large base of support as indicated by the grey area in Figure 2.14. We can calculate the BoS simply as the area, i.e. width × length, of the contacting surface.

The box is a simple example; however, what about the BoS for more complex shapes like the human body? While standing with feet apart the base of support of a human is defined by the shaded areas in Figure 2.15.

As you can see from the footprint diagrams the base of support does not have to be all in contact with the supporting surface; rather it is the area defined by the perimeter round all the points in contact. Think of the 'feet' of the Eiffel Tower. It wouldn't be as much fun if you couldn't walk under the tower but the fact that the actual contact points are relatively small doesn't alter its stability because the area between the points is what matters. Take another example: if we look at a chair (Fig. 2.16) the points in contact are relatively small; however, the base of support is actually quite large.

pushed out of an important position, for example a goalkeeper being jostled out of the way during a corner kick in a game of soccer. A more stable body is less likely to fall or be displaced from a push or pull. So how can you improve stability?

The previous section on mass and CoM is very important for understanding a body's stability. We need to know where a body's CoM is located; however, we also need to know about its base of support

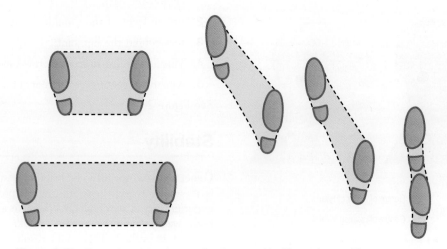

Figure 2.15 • Base of support of a standing human with different feet position.

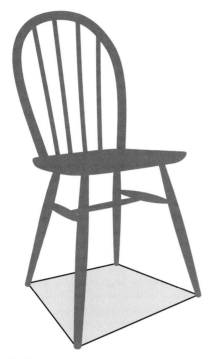

Figure 2.16 • Base of support of a chair.

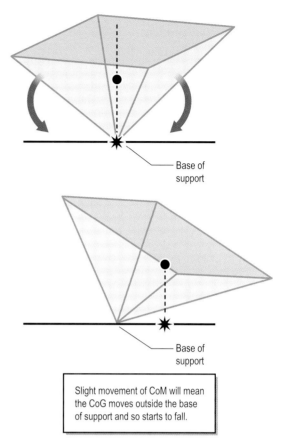

Slight movement of CoM will mean the CoG moves outside the base of support and so starts to fall.

Figure 2.18 • Inverted pyramid showing centre of mass, centre of gravity and base of support.

A body is considered stable if its CoM lies within the base of support. Well, actually it's the centre of gravity (CoG), which is slightly different and easily confused. If you take a line vertically down from the CoM (if you remember, this is the line of gravity) then the point where this line meets the ground is the CoG. A stable body has the CoG within the base of support. Think of the Egyptian pyramids (Fig. 2.17): they are pretty stable structures with the CoG well within the BoS.

But what if we turn an Egyptian pyramid upside down? It's still stable but only if we manage to balance the CoM directly above the rather small base of support. You can see how this pyramid could easily become unstable; i.e. it wouldn't take much for it to topple (see Fig. 2.18).

A body's stability (you could also use the word equilibrium) could be described as one of three types:

1. Unstable—if pushed, a body will move and continue to move until it reaches a stable position;

2. Neutral stability—if pushed, a body will move to a new position where it will remain; and

3. Stable—if pushed, a body will move then return to its original position.

Now once you have made a cone (see Further Information 2.3 for simple quick instructions) try to position it in the three types of equilibrium; see Figure 2.19.

💿 CD-ROM activity 2.4: Stability

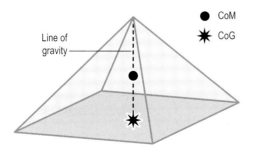

● CoM
✶ CoG

Figure 2.17 • Pyramid showing centre of mass, centre of gravity and base of support.

Further Information Box 2.3

How to make a paper cone

Get a piece of A4 paper, a small plate, pencil, sticky tape and scissors.

Use the plate to draw a circle on the paper; the bigger the circle, the bigger the cone. Now carefully cut out the circle, and fold it in half and then half again so you have a pizza slice. Open out your circle so you can see the four triangles and cut one of them out. Now bring the two edges you have cut together and overlap them (the more you overlap the narrower the cone) so that you have a cone. Tape the ends down.

Further Information Box 2.4

The Belarussian Aleksandr Bendikov incredibly managed to balance 783 dominoes on top of a single domino, so that it was basically an upside down pyramid. Unbelievably this structure stood for a couple of days in his apartment before the media came to witness it. It couldn't have been an easy wait and I don't suppose he was very tolerant of anyone slamming the door. Why don't you try to build one for yourself: all you need is 800 or so dominoes, a flat surface, plenty of time to kill and a very steady hand.

Practical Activity Box 2.4

Have another look at Figure 2.8. You have already identified the CoM; now define the base support so that you have some indication of stability. Is the CoG within the BoS? How close is the CoG to the borders of the BoS? Think about how easy it would be for the person to become destabilized and what direction of push would they be most vulnerable to.

Local and general stability

Because we are made of multiple segments you could have a situation where there is instability between a couple of segments but overall the body is stable. The spine gives us a good illustration of this difference, between intrinsic and extrinsic stability. The spine consists of 12 segments stacked on top of each other with their characteristic three curves. Let's look at the spine from the back and consider each segment at a time (see Fig. 2.20). The CoM of the top segment is located (more or less) at its centre and lies nicely within the base of support of the supporting surface, i.e. the top surface of the next surface down. At this level the segment is stable, locally and intrinsically. In a well-aligned spine this situation carries on all the way down to the bottom segment which in turn rests on the sacrum. The structure of each individual intervertebral segment and the way they are stacked on top of each other confers a great deal of intrinsic stability to the spine; stripped of all its muscles the spine would still be regarded as an intrinsically stable structure.

Now consider a small lateral shift in one of the segments, the second one down. Although overall (extrinsically) the spine is still stable, because the overall CoM still lies within the base of support, the second segment down is outwith its base of support and is therefore intrinsically unstable.

Any local instability, even if it does not affect overall stability, still requires a local solution. If you were an engineer and this was a tower you might bolt some plates or extra cables over the local instability; otherwise it could cause the tower to fall because that individual will eventually break because of the stress. In the body additional muscle work and perhaps some adaptation of other tissues (ligaments and capsule) prevent the segment from

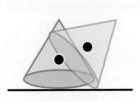 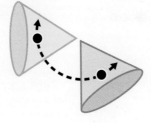 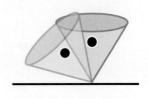

Stable   Neutral stabilty   Unstable

Figure 2.19 • Three categories of stability; stable, neutral and unstable.

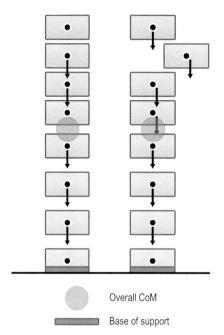

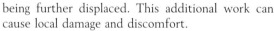

Overall CoM

Base of support

Figure 2.20 • Intrinsic and extrinsic stability.

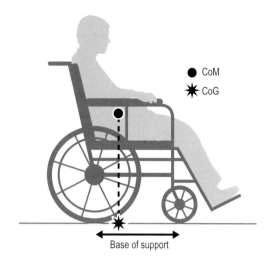

● CoM

✱ CoG

Base of support

Figure 2.21 • Stability of a wheelchair user.

being further displaced. This additional work can cause local damage and discomfort.

The stability of a body is a fundamental design consideration in the construction of many structures from simple furniture to high storey buildings. Wheelchairs are no exception. It's pretty important that a wheelchair remains stable despite being pushed backwards and forwards, bumped up/down kerbs, moved up and down slopes and manoeuvred around obstacles. It is also important to know whether the stability is affected by changes in the user's body mass (e.g. putting a lot of weight on) or the attachment of a rucksack over the back.

So how are wheelchairs designed for maximal stability? First let's just look at a standard wheelchair and identify the CoM, CoG and BoS. When estimating CoM you should consider the person and wheelchair as a single unit. The BoS is defined by the parts in contact with the ground, i.e. front wheels and back wheels.

As you can see (Fig. 2.21), on a flat surface the wheelchair is stable with the CoG well within the base of support. However, what happens if the wheelchair goes up a slope? (Fig. 2.22)

This is obviously a precarious situation, with the CoG close to, if not past, the rear boundary of the BoS. What can you do to reduce the risk of the chair (and occupant) tipping backwards?

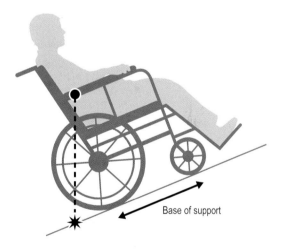

Base of support

The CoG is now behind the base of support, the wheelchair and occupant are therefore unstable and in danger of tipping backwards

Figure 2.22 • Stability of a wheelchair user going up a slope.

• Lean forwards?
• Increase the BoS at the back?

Both options can increase stability. Leaning forwards, of course, moves the CoM forwards and therefore returns the CoG within the BoS again.

Increasing the BoS at the back is achieved with wheelchairs that have their back wheels fixed further back, thereby increasing the BoS (this does, however, make them a little less manoeuvrable). Many wheelchairs have included small stabilizer wheels at the back; these are designed so that they come in contact with the ground with the slightest posterior tip (Fig. 2.23). This contact moves the BoS backwards so that the CoG is again within the BoS, i.e. it stabilizes. This is a bit like moving your foot back to keep balanced when someone pushes you from the front, changing your BoS to accommodate a new CoG position.

Can you think of any other situations when a wheelchair may become unstable?

- What would happen when moving down a slope?
- What about hanging a rucksack on the handles at the back?
- Or how about if the occupant becomes a lower-limb amputee?

Answers are in Appendix 2.

Of course, we have just looked at wheelchair stability from one perspective, i.e. forwards and backwards. It doesn't need me to tell you that the wheelchair can be unstable from side to side as well (see Further Information 2.5). The same kind of analysis that we applied for the side view can be applied for the front/back view. How might side-to-side stability of the wheelchair be compromised?

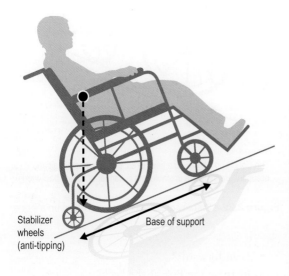

Figure 2.23 • Stabilizer wheels to prevent tipping.

Stabilizer wheels (anti-tipping)

Base of support

> ### Further Information Box 2.5
>
> The sports of wheelchair basketball and rugby involve a lot of potentially destabilizing collisions and rapid accelerations. To minimize the risk of tipping over (difficult to play when you are rooted to the ground) the wheels in these wheelchairs are angled out to increase the width of the BoS, conferring greater stability on the wheelchair and occupant, particularly from the side.

Standing balance

Being upright has produced some excellent outcomes for humans: seeing over walls, freedom to use your hands and skipping, but it has also made us fairly unstable. When you think about it, since we decided to become bipedal, the human body is quite unstable, which is one of the reasons we have such a big problem with falling in the elderly. After all, you do not see many dogs falling over. Becoming upright has moved our CoM much further away from our BoS. Now it can easily (and often does) move outside the BoS. With this arrangement, we have been likened to an upside-down pendulum (like a metronome—see CD-ROM activity 1.2), our mass swaying back and forward and side to side over a relatively small fixed point (our feet); try Practical Activity 2.5.

If we look at the body from the side we can see how this swinging pendulum develops (see Fig. 2.24). Imagine the CoM moved forwards a little; for example you moved both your arms in front of you. With the

> ### Practical Activity Box 2.5
>
> Stand up and close your eyes (make sure you have a clear space around you and don't try this if you have a problem with your balance) and feel yourself gently sway. It is like a tree swaying in a gently breeze. But why don't you just stand still?
>
> As a living organism there are systems constantly at work: your lungs expand, your heart beats and blood gushes round your body and there are constant fluctuations in your body mass. These movements cause the body's CoM to move a little, which is counterbalanced by muscle activity, a little contraction here, another there to dampen any movements of the CoM. Before you know it you are swaying.

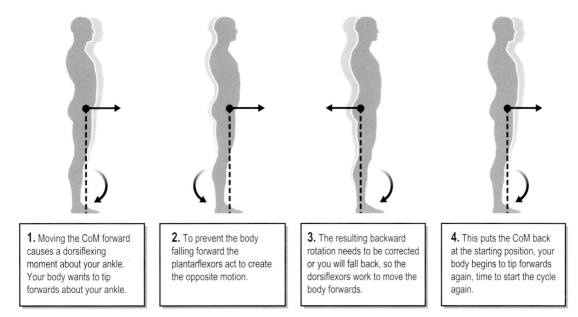

1. Moving the CoM forward causes a dorsiflexing moment about your ankle. Your body wants to tip forwards about your ankle.

2. To prevent the body falling forward the plantarflexors act to create the opposite motion.

3. The resulting backward rotation needs to be corrected or you will fall back, so the dorsiflexors work to move the body forwards.

4. This puts the CoM back at the starting position, your body begins to tip forwards again, time to start the cycle again.

Figure 2.24 • Inverted pendulum.

CoM moving forwards the line of gravity is further in front of your ankle, creating a moment that will bend (dorsiflex) your foot. If left unchecked this moment will mean the whole body will begin rotating forwards. Try it if you like. Stand up and put both arms in front of you, you should feel yourself starting to fall forwards. If you can't feel anything you may be too tense, for this to work you have to be pretty relaxed and in tune with your body. If you do start to fall forwards you only have a short period of time for your body to respond because, powered by gravity, it has started to accelerate towards the ground. Of course your body reacts quickly by creating a counter moment to rotate your body backwards. This is achieved through contraction of the ankle plantarflexors (calf muscles) which rotate your leg, and consequently the rest of the body, backwards. Unfortunately this means your CoM is accelerating backwards, and unless there is another muscle action the body will fall backwards. If you don't believe me why not try it yourself.

Stand up and contract your plantarflexors (press your toes down into the ground—so that your heels lift momentarily). You should feel yourself moving backwards. So yet again the body has to produce a corrective force to make you rotate forwards again. How will this be produced? Step forward the heroic tibialis anterior (the muscle that brings your foot towards your lower leg, a movement known as

dorsiflexion). Practically single-handedly this muscle pulls the body forward again. Again, try it if you like, stand up and quickly pull your toes (both sides) up in the air (a reasonable distance) so that only your heels are on the ground, then immediately let them drop down again. Following this movement you should start to feel your body move forward. So now we are back at the start again with the CoM rocking forwards; the pendulum starts its swing again. This model of balance was first proposed by David Winter, one of the pioneers of biomechanics.

This back and forward rocking movement about your ankle, controlled by the dorsiflexors and plantarflexors, has been called the ankle strategy. It has been suggested that as you get older this strategy for controlling balance is not so effective due to a decrease in the speed that your nerves carry information from your brain to your muscles. Basically the muscles are too far away for an older person to use them quickly enough to react to changes in body position. When this happens, the muscles about the hip are used to move the body forwards and back; this has been called, oddly enough, the hip strategy. The hip strategy is also used if a large shift in the body's CoM is required, for example if you are pushed, with a largish force from the front or back.

Despite our inherent instability humans accomplish some incredible feats of balance. Consider one of the most spectacular circus acts, walking

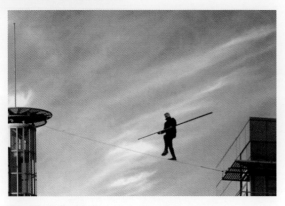

Figure 2.25 • Walking along the high wire.

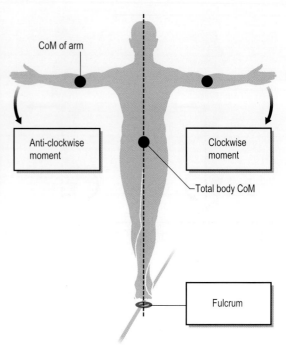

Figure 2.26 • Using equilibrium of moments to perform the high wire act.

along the high wire. During high wire balancing acts (see Fig. 2.25) the BoS is not only small and narrow (the width of the BoS will be essentially the width of the wire) it also moves, really nasty. Lateral (side-to-side) stability is crucial. The acrobat will need to absolutely limit lateral movement and if it does occur, to respond quickly enough to correct the movement before it's too late. They don't have time for an inverted pendulum because that takes too long. One thing that all tight rope or high wire acrobats do is that they all seem to either carry something (usually this is a pole held horizontally but sometimes an umbrella) or hold their arms out to the side. Why is this? Try Practical Activity 2.6; it might give you some clues!

Holding the pole means there is more mass distributed away from the pivot point. This creates moments about the central axis (if you imagine a line up from the pivot point dividing the body, see Fig. 2.26) of the body. These moments can be used to quickly create accelerations of the body, correcting any destabilizing movement, a quick flick of the pole

producing a rapid change in the lateral rotation of the body. There is also a slowing down effect caused by moving mass outwards from the pivot point. This is a bit like making the beam of a seesaw longer so that it takes longer to rotate when a force is applied. We'll talk more about rotation in Chapter 4.

Some tight rope artists hold a pole which is bent downwards. What do you think is the advantage of this? (See Appendix 2.)

Other primates such as orang-utans employ much the same principle when they walk. They deliberately move their arms out to the side so that they can counterbalance lateral momentum. Next chance you get to go to the zoo, have a look at any walking monkey. Do you think they could walk if their arms were tied to their sides?

Practical Activity Box 2.6

Why not try this balancing act yourself? No, not on a high wire (we don't want any casualties)! Just imagine (or draw) a line on the floor and attempt to walk along it. First do it with your arms pinned to your side then try it with your arms out to the side. Finally try it while holding a pole (an unopened umbrella would be fine) level in both hands in front of you. Hopefully you should have felt steadier the second time and even steadier the last time with possibly less muscle work going on around your ankle.

Further Information Box 2.6

In the late 1800s 'the great Blondin' walked across the Niagara Falls on a tightrope. Although an amazing accomplishment in itself, he attempted to make the spectacle even more entertaining with theatrical twists including carrying his manager (I wonder who was the most frightened) and stopping halfway across to cook a meal!

Now that you have thought a bit about gravity, moments and stability why not have a shot at the Practical Activities 2.7 and 2.8. Try to imagine your CoM location throughout the activities.

Understanding a body's stability by identifying the CoM and BoS (Practical Activity 2.4) is, of course, limited because we have looked at a fairly static situation, a snapshot of their movement. We are constantly moving, changing position, direction and velocity and therefore changing our stability. To illustrate this consider the stability of a sprinter at the beginning of a 100-m race. At the start he has a large BoS (defined by the feet, knees and hands—all the point of contact with the ground) and the CoM (or rather CoG) is clearly within this boundary; see Figure 2.29.

At the start gun, the sprinter lifts his head and *hands* simultaneously; this means the BoS rapidly reduces and moves backwards. The CoM (if you imagine it to lie somewhere around the lower abdomen/upper pelvis) and therefore CoG lies well in front of it. From our discussions and activities on

Practical Activity Box 2.7

To remain standing we need a really well-tuned ability to detect our body position (this is also called kinaesthesia). Take a moment to check out your kinaesthetic awareness. Stand up with a bit of space around you so that you are free of objects on the ground and try the following:

1. Close your eyes. Starting at your head think about each body part. Is your head forward on your neck? Is it slightly tilted? Now move down your body, shoulders, arms, hands, pelvis, etc. and try to build a three-dimensional map of yourself. This ability to locate all your body parts in space is critical to balance, as you will see.

2. Now take your shoes off and stand up again. This time concentrate on your feet. Can you identify which bit under your feet is being squashed the most by your weight: Heels? Instep? Toes?

3. OK, now that you have located the area of most pressure under your feet, start to move your body around (without moving your feet). First, slowly lean your trunk forwards until you feel the pressure under your feet move forwards to your toes. Think about your legs and try to identify which structures in your body are being stressed. Can you feel any muscles working harder? This is basically the inverted pendulum we talked about before; see Figure 2.27.

4. Now, go back to normal standing and, without changing anything else, move your arms forwards, starting a little then reaching further forward. How does this change your stability and why?

5. Now remembering to keep your eyes closed lean your trunk backwards. This time you should feel the centre of pressure move back. Unfortunately, you don't have much BoS in this direction so you

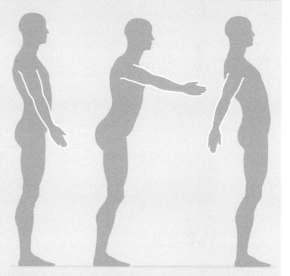

Figure 2.27 • Feeling your balance, practical activity 2.7.

can quickly come to the edge of your stability. Before you reach the point when you have to take a step back, move your arms forwards. Like the last experiment have a think about the movement of your CoM in relationship to your BoS and why the forward movement of your arms was helpful. Do you think it would matter if you moved your arms forwards slowly or quickly?

Once you have done these experiments, why don't you try to move just a small part of your body, e.g. bending elbow and see if it changes the position of the pressure under your feet? You will need very good kinaesthetic awareness for this!

There is an animated version of this showing how the force vector moves about: CD-ROM activity 2.5

Practical Activity Box 2.8

Try this fun activity based around stability and gravitational moments.

Kneel down on the floor and put your hands behind your back. Just as a precaution put a pillow on the ground about a meter in front of you. Now bend down to lightly touch your nose onto the ground just in front of your knees and straighten up, quite easy. Now try to touch the ground further and further away. Sooner or later you will get to a point when you are no longer able to straighten up. Compare your distance with your friends and then try to work out why some people can go further than others. Is there a gender difference?

The first time you did it was easy (relatively) because your CoM was not creating a very large moment. In fact your CoM was probably directly above the knee joint (which is where the body is pivoting) and just a little in front of your hip (so a small flexor moment was created). The next time your CoM was further forwards, creating a larger hip flexor moment and introducing a knee extensor moment. Basically the weight of your trunk/head/arms was rotating your thigh forwards. To prevent you falling forwards you create a counter moment—hip extensor and knee flexor moment—by contracting your hip extensors (gluteus maximus and hamstrings) and knee flexors (hamstrings). If you put your hands on the back of your thigh during the movement you would feel a lot of muscle work. Now the effect this muscle activity has on your lower leg is to lift it up (knee bends). This is unavoidable and just adds to your problems by moving the CoM further forwards and reducing your BoS. You might say you have reached the tipping point, which is why you need the pillow.

Try the same thing again and this time get someone to hold your feet down, you will find that with a stable fixed point the moments created by your hip extensors and knee flexors will allow you to reach further forwards.

Right, did you work out why some of your friends managed to do this better than others? It's all to do with how your mass is distributed. Those of you with more mass higher up in your body, e.g. large muscles in your arms and upper body, will find the task more difficult because when you bend forwards you create a larger flexing moment.

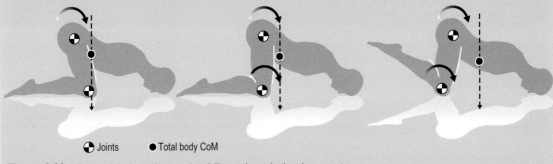

⊕ Joints   ● Total body CoM

Figure 2.28 • Fun activity based around stability and gravitational moments.

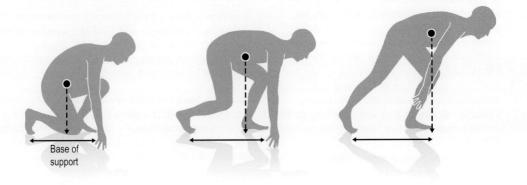

Base of support

Figure 2.29 • Sprint start.

stability we would expect the athlete to fall flat on their face. Although this would probably be very funny, it doesn't happen. So *why* doesn't the athlete fall?

You may already know the answer but if you don't try this activity: Stand up from your chair. Sit back down and do it again but this time do it much slower. Difficult? I am guessing here but you probably fell back down onto the chair the second time. When you performed the movement at normal speed there was a theoretical possibility that you might fall (destabilize) because the body travels through an unstable position between the point when you come off the chair until you are upright. However, because you performed the movement at speed you were able to keep the time spent in this period to a minimum and also the existing forward momentum counteracted the gravitational moments pushing you back down towards the chair.

Try the movement again and attempt to stop at the moment of lift off, look at your BoS and then estimate where (more or less) your CoM is located. The reason you fall back is that the CoM is behind your BoS, which consists only of your feet. Performing the movement at speed means the body gets to the new BoS without destabilizing. Is there anything you could do to improve your stability if, for some reason, you had to perform the movement slowly? What about your foot position (BoS)? Try it yourself. Perform the movement slowly with different foot positions.

There is more information on the sit to stand and stability movement on the CD-ROM; see activity 2.6.

So getting back to the sprinter. The sit to stand experiment should have given you the answer. The sprinter is momentarily unstable as he leaves the blocks but his speed moves his CoM over the new BoS (his feet) before he has a chance to fall, although his feet must move pretty quickly to create the new BoS.

Even during normal walking the body will move in and out of unstable positions. Just before you put your foot down to strike the ground where is your CoM? And where is your BoS? So how would you describe your stability at this point? No wonder walking has been described as a series of falls narrowly averted; this becomes all the more obvious when you watch a toddler learn this very human skill.

So, a body can be theoretically unstable at different points during a movement provided it is moving towards the next BoS quickly enough. There are many other examples when the body is 'theoretically' unstable but the person does not fall. Can you think of any more?

What you need to remember from all that

So, gravity pulls us (speaking as bits of mass) to the centre of the Earth, and is the main force we must contend with. The size of this downward force is a product of our mass (the amount of stuff in our body) and the acceleration of gravity (9.81 m/s/s). This is what is measured when you stand on bathroom scales. Even if our mass remains constant our weight could change if we change the vertical accelerations acting on our body, e.g. going to the Moon or even bouncing up and down. The CoM is a single point that represents all the mass in a body; in quiet standing it is positioned within the pelvis.

Gravity can be considered to act at the CoM of each body segment; this may cause gravitational moments depending on how the limb is positioned.

The stability of a body is determined by the relationship between the BoS and position of the total body CoM. The body may be technically unstable but not fall provided it is moving towards a stable situation. We have also found out how wheelchairs are designed for stability and why high wire walkers use umbrellas to balance.

Chapter Three

3

Force Analysis: Graphs and Maths

What you will learn about in this chapter

1. How to combine forces;
2. How to resolve forces;
3. What happens when force is applied at an angle;
4. How to measure force; and
5. How to use trigonometry to analyse force.

Words you will come across

Resultant, components of force, resolution, force couple, trigonometry, forceplate.

Up to now, we have really only considered a single force at a time, one vector, one arrow on the graph. How easy is that! In our body we have around 700 skeletal muscles, each capable of generating individual force vectors, lots and lots of arrows. Some muscles pass over two joints and so are capable of generating more than one moment at a time. Then of course there are the ligaments which change the direction of a muscle's pull (more on this in Chapter 5) and not forgetting all the external forces that act on us. Performing daily activities means we must contend with lots of external forces. This may be the contact forces with the ground or the weight of a handbag on our shoulder. To understand human movement and posture we need to be able to analyse the action of lots of forces all acting at the same time, some opposing each other, some helping each other. Let's take the first step in this understanding by looking at two forces.

How do forces combine?

The useful thing about force, as you will recall from Chapter 1, is that being a vector you can draw them as arrows and add them together. Let's take a simple example. Two men are pushing a car. The first man, Kenny, pushes in a straight line from left to right with a force of 100 N, the second man, Eddy, pushes with a force of 80 N. To get the combined force (this is also called the **resultant**) we simply add the two arrows together (Fig. 3.1).

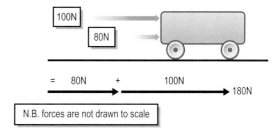

Figure 3.1 • Two forces pushing a car.

That seems pretty straightforward and it would be exactly the same if more people came along. Now, as we know there is a force acting against Kenny and Eddy (otherwise, it would be a pretty easy task), which is the force of friction (which we will talk more about in Chapter 4). If we say that this force has a value of 60 N, this means that the forces acting on the car are shown in Figure 3.2.

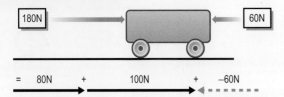

Figure 3.2 • Two forces acting in opposite directions.

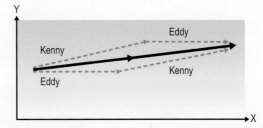

Figure 3.4 • Parallelogram of forces.

This time because one force is acting against the other it has a negative value (remember the reference frames in Chapter 1), so we subtract it, or rather add the negative value, which means the same thing, to get the resultant force. This is the same as

80 N + 100 N – 60 N = 120 N

In the examples so far we have used forces which are applied at right angles to the object (straight at it) but this is rarely the case either in the physical environment or within our bodies. To understand forces acting at an angle let's continue with the car pushing.

Kenny's right hand begins to hurt after pushing for so long so now he only pushes with his left hand; consequently his force changes direction a little (but still with the same magnitude). Now he is pushing at a 25° angle from the horizontal but steady Eddy continues to push straight. To understand how this affects the resulting force you can still add the forces together, remembering to maintain the same angles (Fig. 3.3).

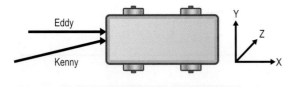

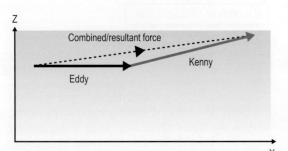

Note that the "vertical" is Z, this is because we are viewing the car from above, so the vertical axis represents side to side movement

Figure 3.3 • Adding forces at angles. This time you are looking at the car from the air.

To understand the effect these two pushes have on the car (you could probably guess but it's good to see how we can accurately calculate the resulting force) we can combine them by adding one to another (nose to tail). The resultant (dotted line) is the connecting line between starting point and end of the two combined force vectors.

This is also known as the parallelogram of forces because you can construct a parallelogram (a figure of four sides where opposite sides are parallel) using the two forces for both sides. The resultant then just joins up the angle at the start with the one at the end (Fig. 3.4).

As well as joining forces together we can also take them apart. It's just the reverse of combining (I probably didn't need to say that). Instead of two people pushing the car let's say we had one—Barry, who pushes the car at an angle. Now the push Barry creates on the car (dotted arrow in Fig. 3.5, F1) could have been achieved by a number of different combinations. From the diagrams in Figure 3.5, choose the combinations which could provide the same push as Barry. See Appendix 3 for answer.

What we are saying here is that we could replace Barry with two smaller forces applied at different angles. For ease of calculation it is simplest to replace Barry with forces that act at right angles to each other. That way we can use trigonometry to calculate their size and direction (more of this later).

If you didn't understand the car example let's try something you can do yourself. Go over to a table, chair or anything really that you can push across the floor (something on wheels would be good, just make sure there is nothing breakable on top before you push). Now push it in the same manner as shown in Figure 3.6, i.e. push down and forward.

Because you are pushing the object at an angle the force you apply could be replaced by a combination of a horizontal/forward push and a vertical/downward push (dotted arrows in Fig. 3.6), depending on the angle of application. You are basically pushing down

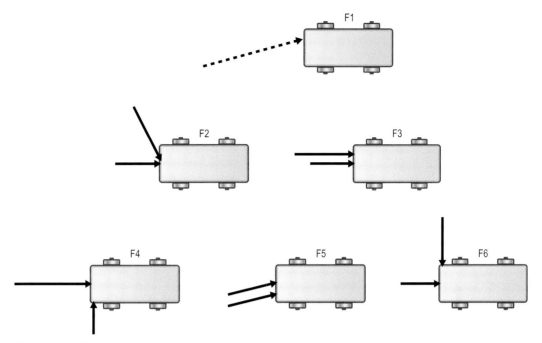

Figure 3.5 • Which combination of forces is correct?

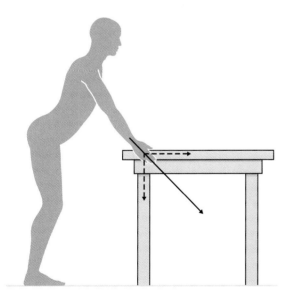

Figure 3.6 • Pushing table.

and forwards. Importantly these two **components of the force** will act at right angles to each other. From this breaking down of forces we can see that only part of the applied force (the horizontal component) will cause the forward motion of the table and that the vertical part does not contribute towards the forward motion. In fact it will make matters worse because it increases the force of friction acting in the opposite

direction—more on this in Chapter 4. So it would be best, of course, to apply the force without any vertical component (see Fig. 3.7).

That's enough pushing of things around. Let's get back to the human body.

Two thigh muscles pull on the patella (knee cap if you haven't covered this in an anatomy class), the vastus medialis and vastus lateralis (there are two other muscles involved but let's keep it simple for now; see Fig. 3.8). We can add the two muscle forcus together, just like Kenny and Eddy (remembering to add nose to tail!), to see the resultant. Remember that the length of the arrow represents the size of the muscle's pull provided you have kept the same scale throughout, of course.

You can probably guess just by looking at the arrows what the resultant force will look like but this is a useful exercise, particularly when things become more complicated. From these two muscle forces we get a resultant (or combined) force that acts to pull the patella up and to the right. This is not a great idea as the patella runs along a kind of groove on the femur (strangely enough this is called the femoral groove). Poor contact between the patella and the femur could lead to local inflammation, pain, swelling, etc., so what can you do to make sure the patella is pulled directly up and not over to one side?

Answer is in Appendix 3.

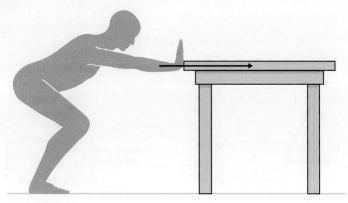

Figure 3.7 • Applying the force horizontally.

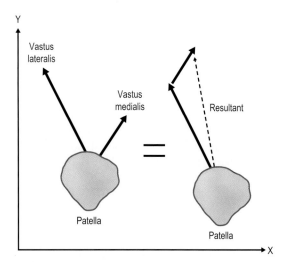

Figure 3.8 • Muscle pull on patella.

The Q angle and knee pain

In fact, it has been speculated by physiotherapists, podiatrists and sport therapists (among others) that the angle of pull of the quadriceps muscle group (Q angle) is one of the causes of pain around the patella (see Fig. 3.9). It has been suggested that a large angle (>15°) to the long axis of the tibia is a risk factor. Furthermore it has been suggested that the reason female athletes are more prone to this type of problem is because they naturally have a larger angle due to the female pelvis being broader. It should be noted that this is still disputed because no clear evidence has been produced. Indeed the notion that females have a broader pelvis (although this may sound intuitively correct) has not been empirically established. What do you think?

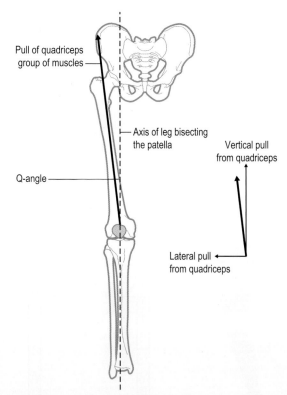

Figure 3.9 • Q angle.

There are, of course, lots of examples of muscles applying their pull on a bone at an angle. For example, let's look at the pull of gluteus medius (GM) on the femur, which is one of the main muscles that lifts your leg out to the side. In Figure 3.10 the black arrow represents the force vector of GM (you will notice that the vector has arrows at both ends; this is just to demonstrate that it can pull in either direction—as all muscles can). For the moment

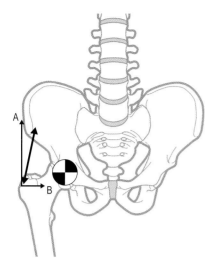

Figure 3.10 • Resolving force of gluteus medius.

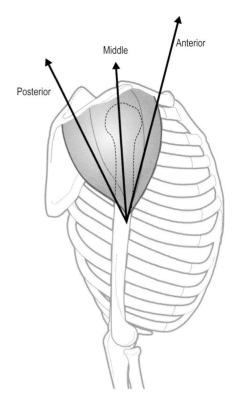

Figure 3.11 • Force of three parts of deltoid.

just consider the pull is on the femur; look at the angle the vector makes with the femur and think about what we have already talked about regarding breaking forces down into their component parts. You should be able to see that the two thinner lines are the result of this pull on the greater trochanter.

The part of the force (A) pulling directly upwards (towards the pelvis) will create the turning force because it is acting at a distance from the joint centre. The other force component (B) is directed downwards towards the joint. The B component may be useful in stabilizing the joint but may also lead to injury because it is compressing the joint together. This is sometimes called the joint reaction force. The joint is designed to cope with these compressions (this will be discussed in more detail in Chapter 7). However, over time these compressions can contribute to erosion of the articular surface and ultimately inflammation of the joint—arthritis.

All our examples so far have been from the lower limbs, so let's move up the body. The deltoid muscle wraps around the outside of your shoulder. This muscle is primarily involved in lifting your arm out to the side (abduction). It is usually regarded as a muscle made up of three parts (front, middle and back) that can work separately or altogether. If all three parts (see Fig. 3.11) were working what would be the result? Remember that in a vector diagram the length of the arrows represents the relative magnitude of the force.

Can you draw in the resultant? Answer is in Appendix 3.

We have been looking at the muscle forces that combine (within our body), but how do external forces combine to act on our body?

When you are standing still you are applying a force down onto the ground (your mass multiplied by the force of gravity—black arrow in Fig. 3.12), which we have already talked about, and the ground applies a force back onto you (grey line in Fig. 3.12) of the same magnitude but in the opposite direction (more on this in Chapter 4). Now the situation during walking is a bit more complicated: you still apply a force onto the ground but this time your force (and consequently the ground's reaction force) is applied at an angle. Take the last point of contact with the ground when you walk, which is usually toe off. To understand the effect this force has we need to break the force down into its component parts (vertical and horizontal (see dotted lines)). From this breakdown we can see that some of the reaction force will be directed horizontally forward (which pushed us forwards) and some vertically up (which lifts our body up).

Have a look at Figure 3.13 and see if you can work out the components of the force based on

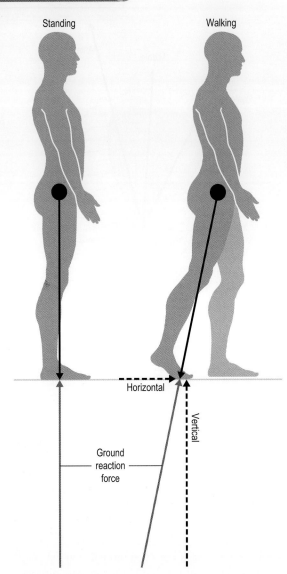

Standing   Walking

Horizontal

Vertical

Ground
reaction
force

Figure 3.12 ● Forces during standing and walking.

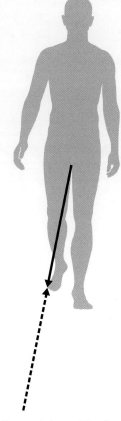

Figure 3.13 ● Forces during walking from front.

the resultant vector and what might be the direction of the resulting motion.

Just like linear (straight) forces we can also add rotational forces (moments). Moments that produce the same motion (clockwise or anti-clockwise) can be added together. If they are opposite to each other they are subtracted. So, for example, imagine two workers using a long lever to help move a boulder (see Fig. 3.14). Man A applies his pull of 90 N

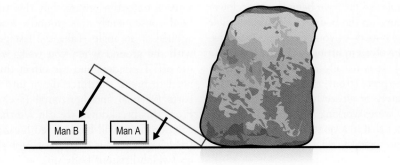

Man B   Man A

Figure 3.14 ● Adding moments

20 cm (0.2 m) from the fulcrum (so a moment of 18 Nm) while man B applies his 75 N at a perpendicular distance of 35 cm (0.35 m) from the fulcrum (so a moment of 26.25 Nm). Because the moments are in the same direction we simply add them to get the net moment (44.25 Nm). If one of them was pushing rather than pulling we would subtract the anti-clockwise motion from the clockwise.

The moments don't have to be applied on the same side as each other to create the same moment. In a **force couple** two (or more) forces are applied in opposite directions and opposite sides of the fulcrum (Fig. 3.15). The result is that they produce the same motion and therefore can be added together. The best illustration of this, from our everyday lives, is the rotating doors typically found at the entrance to big shops. To get into the shop you push one panel of the door, but on the opposite side (trying to get out) is another person pushing on a different pane of the door; the effect is the sum of both your moments. If you try to push on the same panel you will cancel each other out.

There are some examples of this in the human body, e.g. the pull of different parts of the trapezius muscle on the scapula. Perhaps the easiest to visualize is the complementary action of the hamstring muscles pulling the pelvis down at the back and rectus abdominus (the six-pack muscle on your abdomen) pulling the pelvis up at the front.

This example is animated in your CD-ROM—activity 3.1.

Measuring force

One of the tools used in biomechanics to measure force is the forceplate. A forceplate is an example of a transducer, which is a device that changes one type of energy into another; e.g. a solar panel changes light energy into electrical energy and a loudspeaker changes electrical energy into sound. So a force transducer transforms (changes) mechanical energy (a push or pull) into an electrical current. Once the signal has been calibrated, by repeatedly applying forces of known value and measuring the resulting change in current, then unknown forces can be measured by the change in current of the transducer. With careful arrangement of transducers and some mathematics the other components of force (direction, point and angle of application) can be obtained. Two types of force transducer are common:

1. Strain gauges and

2. Piezoelectric crystals (see Further Information Box 3.1).

CD-ROM activity 3.2

Strain gauges are simple devices used to measure force. They are based on strips of metal, e.g. copper, that change their electrical resistance as their length changes, for example when they are stretched (or strained!). Electrogoniometers, for example, are based on strain gauges. Placed across a joint the electrogoniomter will stretch with movement; this change in length causes a change in electrical current. A calibration process determines how much joint movement will create a certain amount of change in current; this is then converted to degrees.

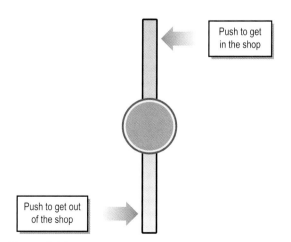

Figure 3.15 • Force couple: rotating doors.

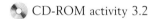
Further Information Box 3.1

The other type of force transducer has come from nature. In the 1880s the Curie brothers (Jacque and Pierre) demonstrated that crystals (like quartz) produce an electrical current when they were mechanically stressed (compressed). This property has been exploited in many devices such as lighters where a small crystal is compressed (when you squeeze the trigger) to produce a spark. The reverse process also works; i.e. if you apply an electrical current to the crystal it vibrates at a certain frequency. This has been used to create ultrasound waves for detection (and diagnostic) equipment as well as for application of therapeutic ultrasound.

Force transducers (crystals or strain gauges) are used in forceplates to measure the amount, direction and location of an applied force.

🔘 CD-ROM activity 3.3

The forceplate consists of a rigid metal platform (this is the surface on which the force will be applied) which sits on top of four columns located approximately underneath its corners and which have force transducers in them. Three transducers are orientated at right angles to each other within the columns. This allows them to pick up force in the different directions (X, Y and Z). The electrical signal is then amplified (volume turned up) and passed onto a personal computer for analysis; see Figure 3.16.

There are four columns in a forceplate so that the location of the force can be calculated. If you stood in the very centre of a square bit of wood that was resting on four weighing scales the readings on all the scales would be the same. If, however, you stood towards the front of the wood the readings on the front two scales would be higher than the back two. So if you only looked at the scales you would know that the person was standing towards the front of the square. The forceplate works in the same way to calculate what is called the centre of pressure. This is the location (or point of application) of the force on the plate; see Figure 3.17.

So basically the forceplate works like a sophisticated bathroom scale. When you stand on a bathroom scale you compress small springs; this change in length of the springs causes (using levers and cogs) a dial to move which has been calibrated to show your weight in kilograms. Because of how scales are designed it doesn't matter (or shouldn't) where you stand, as long as all your weight is on the plate! Because it uses springs which are orientated vertically it can only measure vertical force (which is fine if you are just standing there). The forceplate offers more options: it can locate the exact position of your force on the plate

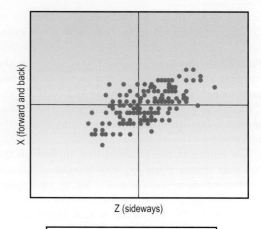

Each dot tells you where the centre of pressure was at a specific moment in time. So if all the dots are close together the person has not wobbled about much.

Figure 3.17 • Centre of pressure measured by a forceplate during normal standing.

(Fig. 3.17), it can calculate the amount of vertical and horizontal force (because the transducers are positioned in different directions; see Fig. 3.16), and the electrical signal from the forceplate can be easily recorded and analysed using a computer. This is quite difficult to do with a bathroom scale as the only 'output' is what you see. The final output from a forceplate has been used to study forces during walking. Have a look at Figure 3.18 and see whether you can interpret the graph. Don't worry if you can't; there is an explanation afterwards. The graph is the recording of force during a single stance phase of gait (i.e. with the foot on the ground).

OK, the explanation of Figure 3.18: I hope you had a shot first, and didn't just jump to this explanation! Let's consider the vertical force first (the dotted line). The graph begins with initial contact (heel strike usually) so you can see this rapid increase in force as the body crashes down onto the forceplate; this force will exceed body weight (we will look at the reasons for this in the next chapter). You may notice a little bump in the graph during this increase; this is called the heel strike transient. It represents a brief reduction in force and is caused by shock absorption (hip, knee and ankle movement on impact). Next comes a drop in vertical force. This is primarily due to the action of the opposite side (mustn't forget we are *bi*-pedal) which isn't on the forceplate. The trailing

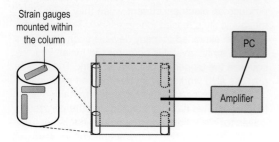

Figure 3.16 • Diagram of a forceplate.

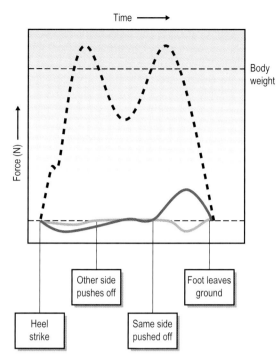

Figure 3.18 • Ground reaction forces during walking (see Further Information Box 3.2).

leg pushes down on the ground (see Fig. 3.12) to push the body up (as well as forward); consequently there is less force acting on the forceplate (you are moving up!).

Further Information Box 3.2

For obvious reasons this graph is also known as the butterfly diagram. For less obvious reasons it is also know as a Pedotti diagram, named after the Italian biomechanist Antonio Pedotti who continues the Italian influence on our understanding of human movement at the Politecnico di Milano.

Following this dip the vertical force increases again to the same level achieved previously. This is again due to the action of the lower limb pushing the person up (and forwards) but this time by the foot resting on the forceplate.

The horizontal force (black line), although nowhere near as large as the vertical, is still interesting. You will see that the force is immediately negative; this is a braking force (that you must overcome to continue moving forwards) applied in front of your centre of mass (CoM) at your forward foot. The direction of this force switches to positive

towards the final third; this is because the body (CoM) is now ahead of the standing foot. Consequently the applied force will be directed backwards on the ground with the reaction force directed forwards to push you forwards onto the next step (a little like walking in Fig. 3.12). How did you get on with that? We will be revisiting force and change in motion in the next chapter so if you found that difficult to follow, don't worry the next chapter should help.

Using mathematics to resolve force

The graphical method of adding forces is easy to follow (hopefully) and has the benefit of being able to show the result. It can be quite difficult, however, to be accurate with this method as it involves a lot of measurements, all of which may fall foul of human error. There is another way of adding force that involves trigonometry. There is nothing terribly difficult about it, but it does put some people off, so we will take it easy in this section. If you really hate this kind of thing, why don't you just glance through it until the summary at the end? You could always try again later.

The whole principle revolves around some special properties of right-angle triangles (two of the sides are placed at 90° to each other), which the ancient Greeks (such as Ptolemy and Pythagoras) worked out two and a half thousand years ago; see Further Information Box 3.3. Thanks to them, in a right-angle triangle with only a few bits of information we can work out all of the triangle's dimensions. For example let's say side A (Fig. 3.19) has a length of 5 cm and there is an angle of 30°. We can work out all the other angles and lengths from these two quantities. For example, we can work out the size of the hypotenuse (longest side in a right-sided triangle) because the sine of 30° is equal to the opposite side divided by the hypotenuse, i.e.:

sine30° = 5/H

Therefore

H = 5/sin30 = 5/0.5 = 10

So the hypotenuse is 10 cm long. We could have also used the cosine rule, which is the relationship between the hypotenuse and the side adjacent to

Further Information Box 3.3

Geometry and mathematics were a bit of an obsession for the ancient Greeks, particularly those living on the Greek islands and Ionia (which is now in modern-day Turkey) in the centuries before Christ. Pythagoras for example lived 2,500 years ago on the Greek island of Samos. He was the leader of the cult the Pythagoreans, who (as well as avoiding eating beans!) believed that the answers to the universe lay in mathematics. He is perhaps most famous for proving the theorem which now bears his name: that the square of the hypotenuse (longest side in a right-sided triangle) is equal to the sum of the squares of the other two sides. Although there is evidence of other cultures knowing this relationship it was Pythagoras who sat down and worked out that it is true for every size of right-angle triangle. He also talked about it a lot.

A couple of hundred years later Ptolemy from Ionia established the sine and cosine laws (as well as the inverse rules) of a right-angle triangle but of course, like many discoveries, these mathematical functions had a previous history in China and India. Before Ptolemy, however, the relationships were documented as a big book of tables. These special relationships in a triangle became known as trigonometry and were a real breakthrough for mathematicians, engineers, builders and architects (not to mention physiotherapists and podiatrists!).

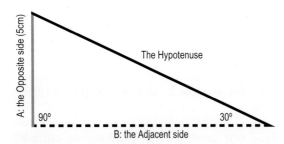

Figure 3.19 • Right-angle triangle.

the known angle (side *B* in Fig. 3.19). It states that the cosine of the angle (30° in our case) is equal to the adjacent divided by the hypotenuse (which we know is 10 cm for our triangle). So:

cosine30° = *A*/10

so

10 × cosine30 = 8.66 cm

So now we know all three sides, but if we only knew two we could calculate the last one using Pythagoras's theorem (see Further Information Box 3.3).

We have talked quite abstractly here. Let's get back to force and biomechanics. Imagine you are pushing a table across a room and the direction of your push is not straight but at an angle (just like in Fig. 3.6). Previously we just drew the components; this time we will use trigonometry.

The push (black line in Fig. 3.20) can be resolved into two components (at right angles to each other), one acting horizontally (black dashed arrow) and the other acting vertically (grey arrow). This is just as we discussed previously. Now if we know the size of the hypotenuse, which in this case we call the resultant, and the angle it is applied to the box then we can work out the other two components exactly.

Let's suggest that the force has a magnitude of 35 N and is applied at the box at an angle of 30° to the horizontal, we can construct a right-sided angle; see Figure 3.21. We can now use the sine rule

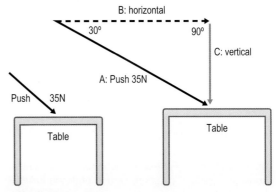

Figure 3.20 • Push on table resolved into components for mathematical analysis.

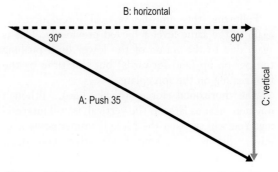

Figure 3.21 • The push viewed as a right-angle triangle.

to calculate the size of the opposite length (which in our case is the vertical component):

sine30° = opposite/hypotenuse (35)

Therefore:

0.5 = opposite (unknown)/35

Therefore:

35 × 0.5 = opposite, i.e. 17.5 N

If we know the hypotenuse and we know the opposite we can calculate the remaining length (horizontal) using Pythagoras's theorem:

Hypotenuse squared = opposite squared + adjacent squared

Therefore:

35^2 = 17.5^2 + adjacent (unknown horizontal component)

Therefore:

35^2 – 17.5^2 = adjacent squared

Therefore:

adjacent squared = 918.75

so the adjacent (horizontal) is the square root of this, i.e. 30.3 N. Therefore, we now know that if we apply a force of 35 N to a box at an angle of 30° to horizontal, it will result in a vertical component of 17.5 N and a horizontal component of 30.3 N.

The relevance here for the human body is that skeletal muscles apply their forces on moving bones, which will inevitably mean that the force is being applied at an angle. Let's consider the pull of the biceps muscle. If the forearm was positioned at 90° to the upper arm then the biceps would apply its force completely vertically, i.e. no resolution; see Figure 3.22.

Now, if the elbow extends (straightens) even by a little, then the angle of pull of the biceps muscle on the forearm will change. When it is no longer being applied at 90° the muscle force is resolved

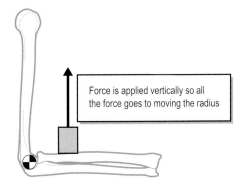

Force is applied vertically so all the force goes to moving the radius

Figure 3.22 • Pull of biceps at an angle.

into vertical and horizontal components. We can use trigonometry again, but we need a few bits of information. The size of the pull, let's say it is 50 N, and the angle of application, let's say 25°, would be sufficient for us to construct a right-sided triangle and apply the cosine or sine laws, see Figures 3.23 and 3.24.

It doesn't take a huge leap of imagination to realize that we can apply this analysis to multiple muscle forces at the same time to work out all the forces involved in a complex problem. This is

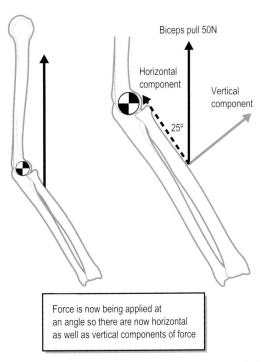

Biceps pull 50N

Horizontal component

Vertical component

25°

Force is now being applied at an angle so there are now horizontal as well as vertical components of force

Figure 3.23 • Resolution of muscle force when applied at an angle.

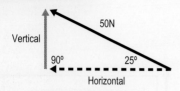

So we can use trigonometry again. We can use the cosine rule to calculate the size of the horizontal force which is the side adjacent to the angle we know (25°).

Cosine of 25° = adjacent/hypotenuse (50N)

Adjacent = Cosine 25 x 50 = 45.3N

Figure 3.24 • Analysing force applied at an angle by using a right sided triangle.

exactly what biomechanists/bioengineers do by constructing free body diagrams where some of the forces and some of the angles are known (e.g. by measuring with a forceplate) and the rest can be calculated with trigonometry. Something for you to look forward to.

What you need to remember from all that

This has been a pretty mathematics-based chapter so it is good to recount the things you must remember.

Forces are vectors, so they can be added nose to tail. Provided the angles and lengths are kept consistent there is no end to the number of forces that can be analysed in this way. Rotational forces can also be added if you know the motions they will cause. As well as adding forces they can be resolved into component parts which act at right angles to each other.

There are different ways of directly measuring force. The forceplate is used for measuring different movements including gait. We examined a Pedotti diagram, so that won't be new to you next time. (It's amazing what you can see in those graphs if you look hard enough!)

Finally we used mathematics or more specifically trigonometry to work out, exactly, what happens when muscle forces are applied at angles.

Chapter Four

Forces and Motion

4

What you will learn about in this chapter

1. What resists movement;
2. How force causes movement;
3. All about momentum, angular and linear;
4. The relationship between impulse and momentum;
5. What pressure is; and
6. What friction is and how it affects motion.

Words you will come across

Newton's laws, inertia, moment of inertia, momentum, impulse, action, reaction, pressure, centre of pressure and friction.

Up to now we have dealt with forces in a static kind of way. All the forces have been balanced, or are in equilibrium if you like. In this chapter we will look more at forces when they are out of balance. This will necessarily feature Isaac Newton's laws of motion. We will consider how movement starts (and stops), how it is controlled and how it is described. We will look at bodies moving in straight lines (linear) and those moving in circular motion (rotation). We will also consider friction and pressure as these are key concepts in understanding force and movement as well as biomechanics in general.

Let's start with a reminder of what a force does. The push or pull of a mechanical force does two things to a body:

1. Produces a change in velocity; this could be magnitude and/or direction because velocity is a vector; and
2. Changes its shape, e.g. lengthening, compressing or distorting (we will find more about this in Chapters 6 and 7).

Of course chances are that both of these will occur to a greater or lesser extent.

Inertia

The way that the motion of a body is affected by a force is enshrined in Newton's three Laws of Motion, which we will get to in a moment. However, it is easier to understand these laws if you consider the body to be rigid; i.e. it won't deform (change shape) when the force is applied.

Let's imagine this rigid body, a brick for example (Fig. 4.1).

The brick is happy where it is and sees no good reason to move. For the brick to move, someone or something is going to have to apply a large enough external force (push or pull). This reluctance to move is a property of all bodies and is called *inertia*. Inertia has been in our scientific knowledge since the experimental work of **Galileo Galilei** almost 400 years ago (see Further Information Box 4.1). In fact inertia comes from the Latin word for laziness and is dependent on the amount of mass a body has. This is a simplification, but the more mass a body has, the more reluctant it is to move. Put another way, to get a big brick moving you need a push bigger than that to move a small one.

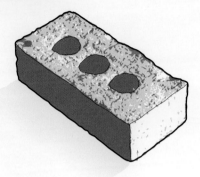

Figure 4.1 • Brick.

Inertia is a key principle in biomechanics but it doesn't just apply to objects sitting at rest. The same principle applies to bodies in motion. Let's consider the brick again; once you apply the push it will move off in the direction of the push. You have changed its velocity. Now that it is moving, it really doesn't want to change again; it's happy moving along at this new velocity, in this direction, forever. Before, it was reluctant to move from rest; now it is reluctant to change from a constant velocity. Rigid bodies can be pretty stubborn! If we want to change its velocity (stop it, slow it down, increase it or change its direction) we will need to apply yet another force.

In reality we know that the brick, once pushed, does not travel in that direction for very long. When you push a brick it might move a couple of reluctant metres before stopping; it certainly doesn't continue moving at a constant velocity forever. This isn't, however, a contradiction to what I have just said. The reason the brick slows down is that another force, **sliding friction** (which we will talk more about later in this chapter), and some resistance caused by moving through air (more on this in Chapter 8) act in the opposite direction to the brick's motion, eventually making it stop. Everything is back in balance again.

What we have just talked about is known as the law of inertia. Although first described by Galileo, it was Isaac Newton who clearly described its relationship with force. Newton wrote:

Every body perseveres in its state of being at rest or of moving uniformly straight forward, except insofar as it is compelled to change its state by force impressed.

Further Information Box 4.1

As we have already discussed, Galileo was not happy with theory; he wanted to test things. Galileo explored the idea of inertia with a simple, yet elegant experiment. He placed balls on curved tracks of varying gradient. The ball, placed at one end of the slope, would roll down the slope (pulled by the force of gravity) and up the other end (slowed down by the pull of gravity) until it reached its original height, theoretically at least (Fig. 4.2A). In this way the balls behaved very similarly to a pendulum. Galileo made smoother and smoother slopes and balls until he found the balls were very close to achieving the same height. Galileo then reduced the gradient of the slope (Fig. 4.2B) and found that the ball would move along the slope until it reached the same height, even though it had to travel a greater distance. This continued as the slope was reduced more and more until it became flat (Fig. 4.2C). At this point, Galileo concluded, the ball would continue to move forever in the same direction. What he had demonstrated was inertia. The fact that the ball doesn't continue, no matter how smooth the slopes are made, is evidence of friction.

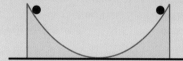

(A) Ball returns to the same height (in a friction-free slope)

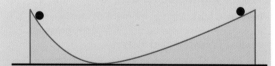

(B) Even if the gradient is altered

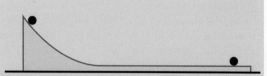

(C) If the gradient were zero (i.e. flat) the ball should continue forever

Figure 4.2 • Galileo's friction-free slopes.

CD-ROM activity 4.1

The experience of being in a rollercoaster is a bit like Galileo's experiment. Once you have been pulled up to the first high point you rush down to the bottom, pulled by gravity, and then up to the next top. In the classic (old-fashioned) rollercoaster each top was a little lower than the previous one. Why do you think this was?

Written in the florid language of the time this is a bit of a mouthful, so we can paraphrase to:

A body continues to maintain its state of rest or of uniform motion unless acted upon by an external unbalanced force.

We will continue to talk about inertia in this chapter as it is a really important and central principle of biomechanics. For simplicity you could just think of it as a reluctance to move or laziness, as Isaac Asimov described it.

One of the important aspects of the law of inertia is that force is **not** required to keep a body in motion (once it has started). You might not think this sounds right, which is what most people thought before Galileo (see Further Information Box 4.1) and Newton. To understand why this is correct you need to understand all the forces involved when an object moves, **friction** and **air resistance** being the main forces that oppose movement. If we could remove these opposing forces then the force we applied to the brick would indeed cause it to move at a constant velocity (and direction) forever.

Moment of inertia

Up to this point we have considered the reluctance of a body to move in a linear direction. Inertia is also an issue if you want to rotate a mass but it's not as simple as how much mass there is. If you want to rotate a lump of mass, such as your leg when walking, then you must overcome its rotational inertia or moment of inertia (a body's resistance to rotation). In a rotating body the distribution of the mass relative to the point about which it is rotating is also a factor. We have talked about it before in Practical Activity 2.3.

The moment of inertia (I) is calculated from the body mass (kg) multiplied by the square of the distance (radius, r) from the point of rotation. For simplicity we can consider the centre of mass (CoM) to be the position of all the bits of mass, which saves us working out the moments of inertia of every particle. This can be summarized as

$I = mr^2$ and is measured in kg/m^2

So, for a point of mass rotating about an origin the further away it is from the centre, the greater its moment of inertia. This is just the principle of

moments restated: the further away from the fulcrum, the harder it is to move.

If you had to push a child in a swing and there were two swings free, one with a long chain and one with a short chain, pushing the child in the short swing would require less push from you. This is because there is less resistance to a rotational force because the mass is distributed closer to the pivot. For the same reason it is easier to swing a flexed leg when you walk than a straight one. However, there is one other major advantage to bending the swinging leg during gait. Have a think what this could be. If you try it out it might become obvious. (See Appendix 4.)

If you are musical you may have come across the mechanical metronome (that little upside-down pendulum that ticks back and forth to help you keep rhythm). To alter the speed of the metronome you slide the counter (lump of mass) either up or down the swinging arm; in other words you alter the moment of inertia of the pendulum. We will talk more about metronomes later when we consider conservation of angular momentum.

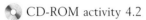 CD-ROM activity 4.2

So, to recap, inertia is the property of a body that resists changes in motion. This is determined by mass when the motion is in straight lines. For rotating bodies it is the mass and how it is distributed relative to the point of rotation that resists rotation.

Linear momentum

Let's get back to the brick which was happy in its sleepy inertia until another force comes along, a push for example. The brick will move in the direction of the applied force provided it is large enough to overcome the brick's inertia. Basically the push has changed the brick's velocity: before it had none and now it is moving at a velocity measured in metres per second (m/s). If a body is moving it has ***momentum***. This is simply the product of its mass (in kg) and its velocity (in metres per second) so the units of momentum are kg/m/s.

We can find plenty of examples of the relationship between momentum and force (in fact, anything that moves would do). For example imagine a game of golf. You lift your club up and swing it down to strike the little white ball. The ball (if you managed to hit it, which I often don't) instantly changes its momentum and travels in the direction of your applied force. If you got this right the ball would have horizontal and vertical momentum as it sails towards its target. Of course, as you know, the ball doesn't fly forever, impeded by air resistance and our old friend gravity, which oppose horizontal and vertical motion respectively. The ball hits the ground and continues to move forwards because it still has some horizontal momentum. The resistance from the grass and perhaps the friction from the ground reduces this momentum until it reaches zero; the ball then stops. Friction and air resistance have opposed the ball's motion, just like Galileo's slopes (see Further Information Box 4.1). One force—the impact of your club—increased the ball's momentum; the opposing forces of gravity, air resistance and friction conspired to reduce this momentum until the ball stopped, close to the pin hopefully.

CD-ROM activity 4.3

The point of all this talk about golf balls is that to **change** a body's momentum—e.g., stop it, start it, speed it up, slow it down or change direction—requires a force (e.g., your push). This is the essence of Newton's Second Law of Motion, the law of acceleration, which we'll cover in more detail a little further on.

Momentum is a vector so we need to state a direction, down, up, east, west, etc., using a common reference frame (see Fig. 1.3). Because we live in a three-dimensional world a body may have momentum in three different directions at the same time. Like any other vector (e.g., force; see Chapter 1) you can combine momentum vectors and you can resolve them into component parts.

CD-ROM activity 4.4

When you are walking you simultaneously have forward, lateral and vertical momentum; behind each direction of momentum is a force. Take the point at the beginning of the swing phase when your trailing leg is about to be brought forward (see Fig. 4.3); during this movement your body (represented by the CoM) moves forward, lifts up and moves laterally towards the opposite standing foot. This momentum is generated by the pushing down action of the leg behind you. Well actually it's the reaction force from the ground that pushes you

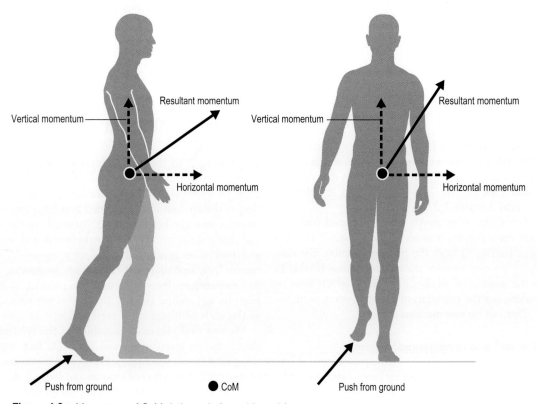

Figure 4.3 • Momentum of CoM during gait: from side and front.

forwards but we don't cover action and reaction until later in this chapter, so keep that bit of knowledge to yourself.

Separating the body's momentum into component parts provides a useful method for analysing a movement because it tells us about the forces acting on the body, their direction and magnitude. Think about the motion of your body during the sit-to-stand movement. The diagram in Figure 4.4 is taken from a movement analysis study that tracked the motion of the CoM during a sit-to-stand movement. The black line represents horizontal momentum and the grey line represents vertical. So you can see the relationship between the two. Horizontal momentum reaches a peak early in the movement due to the rapid trunk flexion created by the turning force of the trunk muscles while still seated. This momentum then reduces rapidly as vertical momentum increases brought about by large moments about the hip and

knee which accelerate the body vertically against gravity, this occurs around about the point when your bottom comes off the seat (seat-off).

The reduction in horizontal momentum around seat-off is clearly important; otherwise you would fall forwards. Try it: stand up from your chair without stopping your forward motion. Your additional step was necessary; otherwise, you would become unstable. So you need to create a force in the opposite direction (a braking force) to reduce this forward momentum, in the same way that friction and resistance reduced the horizontal momentum of the golf ball.

From the graph you can see that around seat-off there is a change in direction of momentum, from predominantly horizontal to predominantly vertical, so as the horizontal momentum reduces vertical increases. This period of the movement has been called momentum transfer because this is exactly

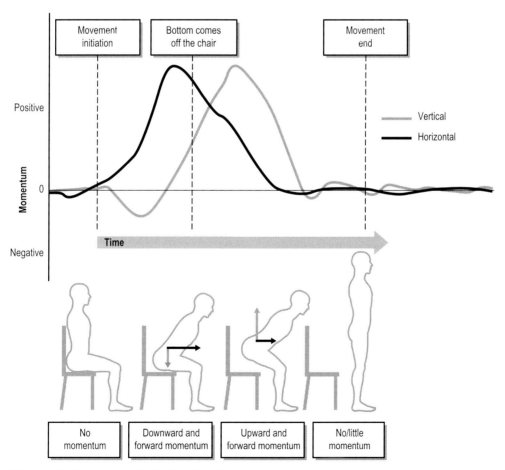

Figure 4.4 • Momentum of CoM during the sit-to-stand movement.

what is happening. The forward motion of the trunk is transferred to vertical motion of the thigh and lower leg.

How do you think this transfer occurs? Answer is in Appendix 4.

Again it is worth remembering that each of these momenta (plural for momentum) and any change in their direction or magnitude is caused by a force.

 CD-ROM activity 4.5

Rotational momentum

In the previous examples of gait and sit to stand we have considered the body's momentum to be directed in straight lines (linear), acting about the CoM. Of course this total body motion is achieved through rotation of the peripheral joints and trunk, the lower limbs in particular. So we really need to understand the momentum of rotating bodies.

As you will recall from Chapter 1 velocity was the rate of change of displacement, how quickly a body moved in a straight line from A to B. If a body is rotating we can still calculate its velocity but this time we use angular displacement, which can be measured in degrees or radians (see Further Information Box 4.2). Let's look at an example to illustrate this: when sprinting the knee flexes (bends) by around 110° (depending on how fast you run), and it does this rapidly. Let's say the movement takes 0.1 s, so angular velocity is change in angular displacement (110°) divided by time (0.1), which is 1,100° per second (pretty fast!). What we have calculated is the velocity of the whole lower leg; things become more complicated when we consider different points on the rotating body. To demonstrate what I mean try following Practical Activity 4.1. You will see that the velocity of mass furthest away from the centre of rotation will be greater than mass next to the centre of rotation, which is why photographs of runners tend to have blurred feet.

Further Information Box 4.2

Radians

A radian is a measure of angular displacement which is equal to $180/\pi$. If you are used to using degrees one radian can be approximated to 57°.

Practical Activity Box 4.1

Get a pencil with a rubber on the end and a paper clip. Undo one of the twists in the paper clip so that you have a long bit which you pierce through the rubber until it comes out the other end (then pull it back so it doesn't protrude). Place the pencil on your desk. Now, if you hold the paper clip you should be able to rotate the pencil about the fixed point, with the paper clip as the axis. Now, with a pen, mark three dots along the length of your pencil more or less evenly spaced (see Fig. 4.5). Imagine these dots represent particles of the pencil so that when you spin the pencil you can see them individually rotate about the origin. You will notice that the dots closest to the centre of rotation move the slowest because they have a smaller circumference to travel through and the ones at the end travel the fastest.

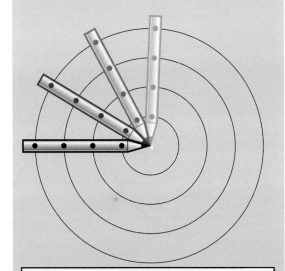

The further away the dot is from the point of rotation the more movement (greater circumference to its journey) it will experience, because the pencil is a rigid body all the dots move at the same time therefore the velocity of the dots towards the outer end will move the fastest.

Figure 4.5 • Rotational momentum with a pencil and paper clip; practical activity 4.1.

Now you may have noticed that I have used the word velocity and not momentum in the last paragraph. This was simply so that you can see how angular velocity is calculated. Of course a rotating body, such as a leg, has mass and therefore momentum.

When a body is rotating it is constantly changing direction, to keep it turning in a circle. A change in direction can only be achieved by a force. This force has two directions which act at right angles to each other (well really three because we live in three dimensions but let's keep it simple). One force causes the forward motion (Fig. 4.6) and the other keeps changing the direction of the body so that it moves in a circle; this force is directed towards the centre (along the string in Practical Activity 4.2), and is called centripetal force. This combination of forces causes the rubber to move in an arc.

Now we talked previously (Chapter 3) about forces being in balance. Therefore the centripetal force needs to have an opposite balancing force; otherwise, the rubber would start coming towards you. This force is called centrifugal and is the opposite (in direction and magnitude) of centripetal. It pushes things out, away from the centre of rotation. Everything is now nicely balanced. You can quite easily feel centrifugal force by trying Practical Activity 4.3. While the centripetal force changes the direction of the rotating body the centrifugal force pushes mass outwards.

We calculated the linear momentum of a body as the product of its mass and its velocity. Rotational momentum, though essentially the same, must consider the distribution of mass so it is calculated

Practical Activity Box 4.2

Get a piece of string (30 cm should do it) and tie your rubber to it. Now go outside to your backyard/ garden and twirl the rubber round and round. Now, as we saw in the previous activity the rubber is going through the same angular displacement as every other point on the string. However, the rubber is travelling through a much bigger distance (greater circumference) so therefore has a greater velocity.

Now let go of the string (being careful to avoid hitting anyone or anything). The rubber moved off in a straight line, right? It didn't continue to move in an arc. This means that the rubber had linear momentum at the time of release, so angular momentum is really just plain old linear momentum. At every moment during the rotation the rubber (mass) has a linear velocity which is directed at right angles to the string. This is well known by discus and hammer throwers who release their projectile at a precise point in the rotation so that the linear velocity is directed up the field. If they get this timing wrong the hammer/discus will move off at an angle which means less distance.

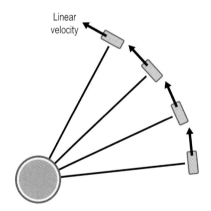

Linear velocity

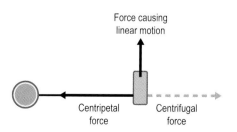

Force causing linear motion

Centripetal force   Centrifugal force

Figure 4.6 • Forces at work during rotation.

Practical Activity Box 4.3

When you run or jog your arm provides some additional momentum (vertically at least). The centre of mass (CoM) of your arm is located somewhere around the elbow so you have to generate sufficient force to overcome its rotational inertia, which comes from the mass multiplied by the distance the CoM is from the shoulder. OK, jog up and down the hall, driveway or wherever and keep your arms straight. Your hands are going through a really big arc of movement compared to your elbows, so there is greater velocity (and of course momentum) at your hands. You may feel more pressure in your hands, which is caused by the centrifugal force (see previous discussion) pushing more blood into your hands as well as stopping blood returning from your hands. You may also feel a little silly.

So what do you do? Of course you bend your elbow. This reduces the moment of inertia so there is less inertia and less muscle to overcome, or if you continue with the same muscle effort your arms will move faster. This is important to keep in time with your leg movement (you may have found this difficult to do with your arms straight).

from the product of the moment of inertia and angular velocity, i.e.

Angular momentum = $I \times \omega$

where I = moment of inertia and ω = angular velocity (typically in radians).

Conservation of angular momentum

I bet you can remember when you were a child, lying on your back on a roundabout and stretching your legs in and out causing the roundabout to slow down and speed up. What you were doing was proving that angular (rotational) momentum is conserved. This is a fundamental principle of moving bodies (linear and angular) that is derived from Newtons Laws of Motion. Quite simply the total momentum of all the objects (ignoring outside interference) will always be the same.

This is what was happening: the roundabout (including yourself) is a rotating body, whose angular momentum is defined by its velocity and moment of inertia. Now when you stretch out your feet you are increasing the moment of inertia by shifting more mass away from the centre of the roundabout (point of rotation). Because angular momentum must be preserved (energy can't just go away—more on this in Chapter 9), this means that to balance the equation angular velocity must decrease. In contrast if you draw you legs back in, the moment of inertia will decrease, meaning angular velocity must increase.

If you can't remember doing this as a child why not experience it now? It will only consolidate your understanding of biomechanics. The idea can also be replicated with your rubber and string (Practical Activity 4.2) by shortening and lengthening the string. Why not try it? But make sure you have plenty of room and no valuables around.

The conservation of rotational momentum is elegantly demonstrated in figure skating when the skaters do those amazing spins on the spot. The velocity of the spin is controlled by the skater moving their arms and legs inwards and outwards. The skater eventually stops the turn by straightening their arms and leg outwards. There are many other examples of rotational momentum being conserved, e.g. the Dad's favourite Christmas toy, Newton's cradle.

There are of course lessons for human movement. Shortening your arms and legs while running increases the rotational velocity simply by reducing the moment of inertia, angular momentum being conserved of course.

Newton's second law: Impulse and momentum

Now we know that if you want to change the way a lump of mass is moving (direction or velocity) you need to apply a large enough force and it will accelerate or decelerate in the direction the force was applied, acceleration being the rate of change of velocity; see Chapter 1 for a reminder. Clear enough I hope; however, the length of time the force is applied also has a bearing on the resulting motion of the lump of mass. This is the nub of Newton's second law which relates impulse to momentum. To understand this let's go back to that stubborn brick.

As you recall we got the brick moving by giving it a push. Now the force from the push must have been applied to the brick over a certain period of time; this time period is critical to the change in momentum of the brick. As any of you who have been taught how to strike a tennis ball or a golf ball should know, you continue to move the racket or club even after impact with the ball. Instructions like 'follow the swing through' may be familiar to you. For example we all know that if we push our brick for a longer period of time it will move away with more velocity.

The reason you do this is to extend the time you are applying the force, to continue the racket swing so that it keeps in contact with the ball for longer. Force applied over a time is called ***impulse*** and this is what causes the change in motion of the body, i.e. **impulse causes a change in momentum**. This relationship is Newton's second law, the law of acceleration, and is described neatly by the formula

Impulse (force × time) = change in momentum

or

$F \times T$ = mass × velocity (after the impulse)
         − mass × velocity (before the impulse)

and

Force =

$$\frac{\text{mass} \times \text{velocity (after)} - \text{mass} \times \text{velocity (before)}}{\text{time}}$$

Because change in velocity divided by time is acceleration this equation for impulse is often simplified to:

Force = mass × acceleration

The relationship between impulse and momentum is an important principle so we are going to conduct a small experiment to make sure you understand; see Practical Activity 4.4.

Let's try some examples based on human movement: Imagine a rugby (or an American football) player running for the score line (see Fig. 4.8). He is big (let's say 100 kg) and fast (let's say he's running at 8 m/s) so he has a lot of momentum (800 kg/m/s)

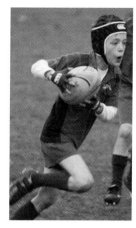

Figure 4.8 • Rugby player running for line.

Practical Activity Box 4.4 (more of a thought experiment really)

There are three ice pucks resting on an ice rink ready for target practice, pucks A, B and C (see Fig. 4.7). They are identical in shape and mass (and distribution of mass).

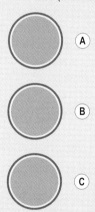

Figure 4.7 • Ice pucks ready to be hit.

Johnny the hotshot striker hits puck A with a force of 35 N; this impact lasts 0.1 s (a snap shot!).

He then comes up to puck B and hits it with less venom (25 N) but increases the duration of impact (0.5 s).

Finally he comes to puck C and decides to wallop it (75 N) and is able to follow through with the stick so that he is in contact for 0.3 s.

Which puck receives the largest impulse and should, therefore, attain the greatest velocity (we can assume the mass doesn't change and there are no other forces acting on it)?

Remember that force × time = change in momentum and that the puck was at rest at the beginning:

For puck A the impulse was 35 N × 0.1 s = 3.5 Ns = $V^2 - V^1$ (zero).

The resulting velocity of puck A as it left the hockey stick was 3.5 m/s.

For puck B the impulse was 25 N × 0.5 s = 12.5 Ns = $V^2 - V^1$ (zero).

The resulting velocity of puck B as it left the hockey stick was 12.5 m/s.

Finally for puck C the impulse was 75 N × 0.3 s = 22.5 Ns = $V^2 - V^1$ (zero).

The resulting velocity of puck C as it left the hockey stick was the greatest at 22.5m/s.

So force (or rather impulse) changes momentum and it's exactly the same for decreasing momentum as it is for increasing it.

🔘 CD-ROM activity 4.6

and he's 15 m from scoring. You are the only player close enough to him to tackle. With every scrap of energy you apply a force of 150 N for 5 s (after which you collapse—beaten), but did you do enough to stop the score?

Let's look at what your impulse (force × time) will do to his momentum:

**Force × time = change in momentum
(mass × V^2 – mass × V^1)**

where V^1 is his velocity before your impulse, and V^2 is his velocity after your impulse (this is what we want to find out). Now the force you apply will be negative as it is against the direction of the other player's motion.

– 150 N × 5 s (your impulse) = (100 × V^2) – (100 × 8)

$$\frac{-750 + 800}{100} = 0.5 \text{ m/s}$$

After your impulse he is still moving! Although at a much slower velocity (0.5 m/s). At this current velocity and with only 15 m to go he will score in 30 s (time = distance divided by velocity = 15/0.5 = 30 s).

What about trying a patient problem?

To get out of a chair an old lady must move her body forwards at a velocity of 4 m/s. Because she weighs 65 kg this means she has a momentum of 260 kg/m/s. Unfortunately, she is a little apprehensive about her balance and so prefers to stop for a moment when she stands up before starting to walk. So she needs to change her momentum from 260 kg/m/s to 0; she can hardly change her mass so she must reduce her velocity. Her muscles contract at the same time to provide a force of −80 N (negative as it is acting in the opposite direction) so how long does it take for her to stop her forward motion?

– 80 N × T(s) = V^2 × 65 kg – V^1(4 m/s) × 65 kg

V^2 is zero (motion stops) so:

**T = – 260 kg/80 N
  = 3.25 s**

This would seem a rather long period of time to decelerate, causing potential problems with stability. What do you think she should do?

Let's end with a rotational problem: An up-and-coming javelin thrower has been given a new javelin

to throw; it is a little heavier (0.5 kg) than the previous one. If he is to reach his usual distance the javelin must be rotated at a velocity of 2.5 radians per second. The CoM of his arm (with javelin) is 0.5 m from shoulder and it weighs around 7 kg. How much angular momentum does he need to create? We are going to ignore any existing momentum due to his run up (makes things easier).

So the mass of the rotating body is 7.5 kg and the radius is 0.5 m (we will assume all the mass is located at the CoM). This means the moment of inertia is:

Mass × radius^2 = 7.5 × 0.25 = 1.875 kg/m/s

If he needs to get achieve a velocity of 2.5 radians per second this means he will need an angular momentum of

Angular momentum = moment of inertia (1.875)

× angular velocity (2.5)

= 3.95 kg/m^{2}s^{-1}

If we knew how long it takes him to throw the javelin we could also work out how much force he needed but I think we have done enough calculating.

I am glad we got to the end of all that rotating. It makes you feel giddy after a while. Let's move away from rotating bodies and consider Newton's third (and final) law of motion.

Newton's third law: Action and reaction

Implicit in our understanding of force and motion is the principle that every action has an equal and opposite reaction, or put another way momentum is always conserved. So for example the centrifugal force was a reaction to the centripetal action when we talked about rotating bodies and the ground reaction force is a reaction to the force we apply to the ground (see Chapter 3). Although mentioned before, it is worth making sure you are clear on the law of **action and reaction.**

Newton described this law:

For a force there is always an equal and opposite reaction: or the forces of two bodies on each other are always equal and are directed in opposite directions.

Or more simply:

For every action there will be an equal and opposite reaction.

It's a simple enough law, but like the previous two laws, absolutely fundamental to our understanding of motion. Let's try a quick experiment: walk over to the wall and put your hands on it with your elbows a little bent, and lean into it as if you are about to do a vertical press up. Now apply a force on the wall by straightening your elbows.

Did the wall move away from you (let's hope not) or change its shape (perhaps imperceptibly)? But you did (or should if you tried hard enough) move a little backwards. This is the reaction force of the wall onto you. You pushed the wall and the wall pushed back on you. If you tried the same experiment in a swimming pool you would feel a greater backward movement because there is less resistance.

Let's consider another example (this time one that moves): two balls colliding, for example in a game of pool. The four ball and the eight ball crash into each other; each applies a push to the other and receives a reaction force (at the same instant) (see Fig. 4.9). The thing to observe is that the interaction between the two balls has resulted in them moving off in opposite directions, but importantly with the same (if we forget friction and air resistance) total momentum. Just like rotating bodies, total momentum in a system (e.g. group of pool balls) is conserved even after a collision.

We should look at a human movement example (we don't want to waste our lives in pool halls).

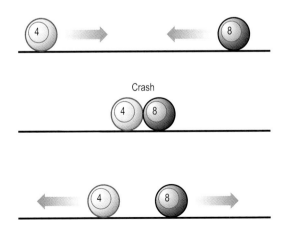

Figure 4.9 • Conservation of momentum after collision between pool balls.

Stand on the bottom step of your stairs and jump down onto the floor. When you land you will apply a large force to the ground; simultaneously the ground applies a force back on you. There has been an equal and opposite exchange of momentum between the two bodies, you and the Earth. The size of the reaction force (acting vertically up) from Earth was enough to stop you dead in your track (changed the momentum drastically); the size of the action force from you to the Earth was enough to change its orbit. Well not really. The size of your force on the Earth is far too trivial to change its momentum, but in theory it did, just a little bit. Perhaps if we all tried a jump at the same time it might be enough to change the Earth's momentum, although I am not sure why we would want to do that!

What you need to remember from that bit

We have covered a lot in the past few pages so it is probably worth recapping a few important points.

- Bodies prefer to stay at rest or move with unchanging velocity (including direction). For objects moving in a straight line this inertia depends on the amount of mass. For rotating bodies inertia depends on the amount of mass **and** where it is distributed relative to the point of rotation. This is called the moment of inertia.
- An unbalanced force applied over a period of time (impulse) alters a body's momentum (stop, start, slow down, speed up and change direction).
- During rotation a body has linear velocity which is constantly changing direction due to a force which pulls the body towards the centre of rotation (centripetal force); this force is balanced by a centrifugal force.
- In a rotating body momentum is conserved: if the moment of inertia changes there is a matching reduction in angular velocity. This principle of conservation also holds true for linear momentum.
- Each time a force is applied (action) there is an equal and opposite reaction force. This means the same as momentum being conserved during an exchange between two (or more) bodies. Although the word reaction

implies some kind of time delay in fact this occurs instantaneously and might be better regarded as an interaction.

Bodies in contact: pressure and friction

When force is applied to a body it is distributed over an area; e.g. when you sit on a chair the combined downward force of your head, arms and trunk presses down onto the chair, but not at one point (which would be a little uncomfortable) instead it is spread over an area, your bottom, back of thighs, back and possibly feet.

Close your eyes for a moment and think about all the points that are in contact with the supporting surface (chair, floor, sofa or whatever you are perched on). Unless you are pretty uncomfortable you should have identified a number of areas (shoulders, back, buttocks, etc.) but not any specific points.

What we are talking about is pressure. Pressure is simply the applied force divided by the surface area. So this could be your force (mass × acceleration of gravity gives you the force) divided by the area of contact, e.g. contact surface of your foot on ground, i.e.:

Pressure = Force (N)/Area (m²)

So the units of pressure are Nm^{-2}.

Consider the old Indian trick of lying down on a bed of nails (see Fig. 4.10). If you try to sit on one nail, of course it will hurt (quite a lot probably so don't try it). But if you spread your mass (and therefore your force) over all the nails, the load on each nail is reduced to the point where it can be tolerated. The more nails the better, i.e. the more points of contact.

This principle of increasing the surface area to decrease pressure is exploited across the animal kingdom. Consider the lowly water skater (or strider): by spreading its legs over as much of the surface area of the water as possible the force at

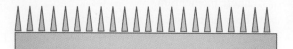

Figure 4.10 ● Pressure to explain bed of nails.

any one point is low enough for it not to break the water surface allowing this delicate insect to glide over the water.

Working in rehabilitation and sports you will come across the effects of pressure on tissue. This could be a life-threatening pressure sore experienced by a bed-bound patient or a blister on your heel from wearing shoes that are too tight. So how does pressure cause such trauma? If you pinch one of your finger nails for a second or two you should see it blanche (go from pink to white). The pressure you applied has pushed the blood away; once you take the pressure off the blood returns and your nail bed returns to a healthy pink colour. Damage occurs when blood is pushed away from tissue for prolonged periods; ultimately the tissue dies because it has been deprived of the oxygen and nutrients it gets from the blood. The resulting dead tissue can become infected with disastrous results. The remedy is not hard to understand: take the pressure off. Practically this can be difficult for some patients who cannot move themselves.

How does understanding pressure help the rehabilitation worker or sports therapist? There are numerous examples:

1. Alleviate pressure in the foot by increasing the contact area with a moulded insole;

2. Apply force in a more comfortable manner, for example by using the palm of your hand when moving and handling a patient, rather than your fingers; and

3. Modify furniture to minimize pressure, e.g. a moulded seat cushion in a wheelchair.

Centre of pressure

The centre of pressure is a term often used by gait analysers, biomechanists and podiatrists among others. You could consider this as the location of the average point of all the pressure applied to a body (we explored this a little in Practical Activity 2.7, p. 31). Stand up (if you haven't completely relaxed on that bed of nails) and consider where your average centre of pressure is (see also Fig. 3.17). You are applying a force more or less evenly across the surface area of both your feet, so the averaged point would be somewhere in the middle, roughly at point A in Figure 4.11. When you are standing nice and quiet this point will coincide with the centre of gravity (point on the ground from the vertical projection

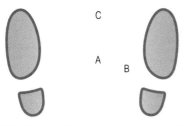

Figure 4.11 • Centre of pressure movement in standing.

of the CoM). Now press harder down on your right leg (but don't move); you are now pressing the ground more on the right side than on the left so the average centre of pressure will move to the right, roughly at point B. What if you pressed your toes down? The centre of pressure would move forwards to point C. You can probably guess the rest, but it is important for you to distinguish between centre of pressure (CoP) and centre of mass or even centre of gravity. Easy to get mixed up with all these centres.

Friction

We have already talked quite a bit about friction as an opposing force in this and previous chapters; it's a difficult thing to avoid when you are talking about movement and one that most people have some understanding of, at least superficially. Hopefully this last section will give you a greater understanding of friction.

Friction is usually regarded as something we don't really want around. Indeed engineers (and rollercoaster designers) spend a lot of their time trying to reduce it to a minimum. It gets in the way of efficient movement. If friction was invited to a party it would sit (unmoving) in the corner, drink all the expensive beer, eat all the pretzels and bore everyone with stories about how it saved a mountaineer from falling to certain death and stopped an old lady slipping. But these stories are not just some drunk's exaggerations: friction can be a force of good. Let me explain.

Friction is a resisting force. It opposes the movement of one body over another, but that doesn't mean it is not useful. Without the friction of a carpet or wooden floor we would find it pretty difficult to stand up, walk or run. We use this resistance to propel ourselves. Imagine trying or live on an ice rink all the time: it would be difficult to get anywhere quickly.

There are three types of friction: the friction within fluids (this will be considered in Chapter 8), the friction between sliding surfaces and the friction from an object rolling over a surface.

Sliding friction, as the name suggests, opposes the sliding motion of a body across another surface. There are two factors involved: first how much the body is pressed against a surface, i.e. its weight (mass × gravity). The heavier an object is, the greater the sliding friction is. This makes sense: a sleeping dog is much easier to push away from the fire than a drunken overweight man. This is only part of the story, however, because the amount of friction is also dependent on the smoothness of the surfaces. It doesn't take me to tell you that the smoother the surface, the easier it is to push something across it. This is called the coefficient of friction and is, essentially, a measure of the roughness of the surface. These two factors cause the relative surfaces to interlock with each other to a greater or lesser extent (try Practical Activity 4.5).

So sliding friction can be represented as:

$$F = \mu \times R$$

where F = force of friction, μ = coefficient of friction (roughness of surface) and R = weight of the object pressing down onto the surface.

Practical Activity Box 4.5

Sliding friction is ubiquitous. Put your finger on the top of the desk and push it along the surface. Depending on the roughness of your finger and the desk surface you should feel some degree of resistance. Now push down harder (increase the R value) and try the movement again. This should be more difficult because you are squeezing the surfaces together more. You will also experience some heat; this is converted from kinetic energy of the movement and isn't particularly useful, unless you use it to warm your hands up by rubbing them together.

Put a paper tissue on the desk and try to do the same thing with the tissue between your finger and the desk. The movement becomes much easier because the interface between the tissue and desk top has a lower coefficient of friction (μ). I am sure you can think of many other ways to reduce the coefficient of friction of the desk top.

Sliding friction is of interest to a range of professionals. Let's looks at a couple of illustrations from healthcare and sport. Nurses need to move dependent patients about their beds. This can be difficult if the patient is large (therefore a large R) and not helped by the sheets which can be ruffled, thereby creating a large coefficient of friction (μ). So what can be done? You can't reduce mass (well not quickly anyway) but you can reduce the coefficient of friction by introducing smoother surfaces such as special sliding sheets (like the tissue in Practical Activity 4.5) or simply tightening the sheets to make them smoother. Talcum powder may be another useful option.

There are many examples of sliding friction in the world of sport. In curling, for example, one or two 'sweepers' are employed to brush the ice immediately in front of the sliding stone to reduce sliding friction, preventing the stone from slowing down as much. The action of the sweepers melts the top layer of ice making it very slippery. On the other hand reduced friction caused by the sweat of volleyball or basketball players needs to be quickly mopped up to prevent injurious slips. Friction has also created challenges and solutions in the workings of the human body.

To improve efficiency the body has attempted to reduce the effect of friction where it can. The sliding up and down of a tendon for example is made easier by wrapping it in a sheath filled with a lubricating fluid which, among other things, reduces the coefficient of friction.

Where sliding friction resists sliding the other main type of friction, rolling friction, resists rolling motion (I probably didn't need to say that!). Rolling resistance is caused by deformation of a circular surface (such as a wheel) as it moves over a flat surface (such as the ground). This deformation basically means more of the moving object (e.g. the wheel) becomes in contact with the ground. There are many factors which affect rolling resistance, for example the shape of the surfaces, the type of material used and the pressure within the material, e.g. in tyres.

Rolling resistance may become a problem for wheelchair users: worn and flat tyres deforming more as it rolls over the ground, creating greater resistance. When it comes to movement, however, sliding friction is a greater consideration.

Finally, although a lack of friction on a surface can predispose to a fall, too much friction can also cause injuries. Consider the graze from falling on rough ground or a blister from your foot moving up and down in an ill-fitting shoe. Even your nipples don't escape friction: jogger's nipple is quite an uncomfortable experience resulting from the friction of your t-shirt as it slides up and down your body.

What you need to remember about friction and pressure

Friction opposes movement. There are three types. In this chapter we considered sliding friction, which has to do with how rough sliding surfaces are and how much they are squeezed together, and rolling friction, which is about circular surfaces rolling over flatter ones, the resistance, in this case, coming from the amount that the surfaces are deformed (think of tyres being pressed onto the road).

Pressure is simply force divided by area and is a consideration for parts of the body under prolonged periods of compression. The centre of pressure is the averaged point of all the pressure points.

5

Work and Machines

What you will learn about in this chapter

1. Concepts of work and power;
2. Machines that perform work;
3. All about levers;
4. Pulleys;
5. Mechanical advantage; and
6. Mechanical efficiency.

Words you will come across

Work, energy, power, levers, pulleys, mechanical advantage, velocity ratio.

Work

In mechanics **work** means that energy has been transferred from one body to another through the application of a force. This means for example that work is done when you throw a baseball (energy moving from your upper limb to the ball) or lift a child or move a patient's leg. But work is also done if you **catch** a baseball (energy moving from the ball to your upper limb), **lower** a child or **resist** a patient's movement. The principle is that energy has moved from one body to another. Work can be calculated as the size of the force multiplied by the distance the body was moved by that force, i.e.:

Work = force × distance

This formula would mean the scientific units are newton metres (Nm), which would cause some confusion with moments, which are also newton metres. Instead the convention is to use joules (J; see Further Information Box 5.1), where 1 J is equivalent to 1 N of force acting over 1 m. Work has magnitude only (no direction is required), so work is a scalar quantity.

Example of work in a straight line

Let's consider a simple situation. You want to push a box 10 m along the ground. To achieve this you need to push with a force of 50 N (see Fig. 5.1).

This would mean that you have performed 500 J of work (50 N × 10 m).

So, provided you know distance and force you can calculate work. The same calculation can be made for rotational movement but we need the

Further Information Box 5.1

Joules

The unit of work (joule) was named after the nineteenth-century British physicist James Prescott Joule. During a period of great discovery, James Joule explored the relationship between heat and work. Through systematic experimentation, firstly with water and latterly with gas, he came up with values for mechanical work being converted into heat; specifically he worked out how much mechanical work (in his classic experiment work was performed by a falling weight) was required to cause a small increase (1°F) in the temperature of a set volume of water.

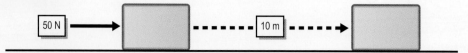

Figure 5.1 • Work.

rotational equivalents of force and distance. Instead of force we have rotational force (moment) and instead of distance we have angular rotation (this is usually measured in radians, which are basically a different way of expressing the degrees of an angle; see Further Information Box 4.2).

Example of angular work

Being safety conscious you decide to tighten up a nut that is holding a table together. You decide to use a spanner (30 cm long) for the job. To turn the spanner you wisely place your hand toward the end of the spanner; let's say 20 cm (0.2 m) from the nut (which will act as the pivot/fulcrum). Of course you push down so that the spanner turns in a clockwise (positive) direction. Let's say that the force you apply with your hand is 80 N and, as we said, it is applied 0.2 m from the nut. This means the moment you apply is 16 Nm (0.2 m × 80 N). So you apply this moment of force until the end of the spanner moves 15 cm and the nut tightens. (We are assuming that the force is applied perpendicular to the spanner throughout.) (see Fig. 5.2).

We can calculate the angle the spanner actually moves through by dividing the angular distance (0.15 m) by radius (0.3 m), which gives us 0.5 radians, a value equivalent to 28.5°.

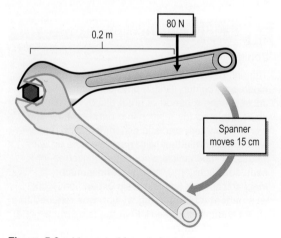

Figure 5.2 • Moment of force to turn a spanner.

The work done is 16 Nm × 0.5 radians = 8 J of work.

Muscles at work

It's about time we got back to looking at muscles. In rising up from a chair the quadriceps muscle group (muscles on the front of your thigh) pull on the femur (which, in this case, is 53 cm in length) to rotate it in a clockwise direction (see Fig. 5.3). To lift your thigh (along with the mass of your trunk, arms and head) the muscle needs to generate a rotational force of 200 Nm (vertical component of force = 500 N multiplied by the perpendicular distance 0.4 m) and the femur moves through an arc of 0.3 m (an angle of 0.75 (0.3 m/0.4 m) radians or 43°). This would mean that 150 J of work (200 Nm × 0.75) were performed by the quadriceps muscles.

Have a look at the following questions, the first of which has been done for you (along with providing some additional information). Then try the other two yourself.

Question 1

A woman is out jogging. For every step she takes her centre of mass lifts by 0.15 m and moves forward by 0.9 m. She weighs 65 kg. To propel her body forward she applies a force of 100 N (this is an estimate based on literature). Calculate the work she does during every step.

Work is performed to move in two directions (there is of course a third direction—side to side—but we will keep it simple). To raise her body 0.15 m she must apply a force greater than the downward force (mass (65 kg) × acceleration (9.81 m/s/s) = 637.65 N), so we can estimate that the force to lift her up is 700 N (62 N greater than the downward force).

So the work done vertically to lift her body against gravity is 105 J (700 N × 0.15 m).

Let's not forget that she is moving forward as well as up. Each step, as we said, takes 100 N

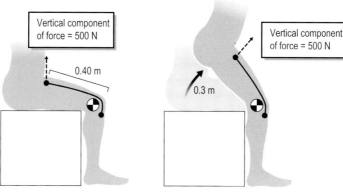

Figure 5.3 • Sit to stand.

of force to displace her forwards (one step) by 0.9 m. So the work done is 100 N × 0.9 = 90 J.

In total then she performs 195 J of work (105 + 90) for each step.

For those of you counting calories this is equivalent to 0.05 cal so twenty steps will expend 1 cal. Just to put it in perspective, a popular nutty chocolate bar contains around 500 cal = 2,000 steps, which, for this woman, would be running for 1800 m (around 1.2 miles).

Of course this is the amount she performs (output) but not the amount her body actually consumes (input) because we are inefficient mechanisms. We will talk about this more later in the chapter. (see Further Information Box 5.2).

Question 2

Calculate the magnitude of force and amount of work in the following situation:

A hoist is used to lift a disabled customer weighing 105 kg into a swimming pool. How much work does the hoist perform when lifting the man 1.7 m up?

Question 3

An angler catches a fish. The fish pulls hard on the end of the line and the angler begins to turn his reel (the pulley mechanism at the end of the rod) to bring

Further Information Box 5.2

External mechanical work versus physiological work measurements

When we performed the calculations earlier we just looked at the displacement of the centre of mass (CoM). This approach does not take account of all the other work which goes on in the body. For example, we must overcome intrinsic joint stiffness and hold body parts steady (e.g. the head and trunk) while other parts move. We even perform work just maintaining balance. Calculating the movement of the CoM also does not consider input from existing potential and kinetic energy from previous steps (Chapter 9 will expand on energy during movement). These calculations, based solely on displacement of CoM, then represent 'external' work. A different approach to calculating work is not to look at output (movement of CoM) but rather input, the energy consumed in performing the action. This can be measured directly by recording physiological markers,

specifically the volume of oxygen consumed during the activity.

There have been numerous papers written on this subject which have compared these two measurements, i.e. the direct cost of all body activity according to the amount of oxygen consumed and the actual mechanical work performed by the body. This comparison provides an estimate of efficiency.

For example research investigations have reported that the efficiency of walking (mechanical output divided by physiological cost) is around 0.25 (i.e. 25% efficiency). This means that for every 100 units of energy used by the body to walk only 25 units have been transferred to mechanical work on moving the body. The remaining 75% has been used for other functions and converted to other forms of energy, heat for example.

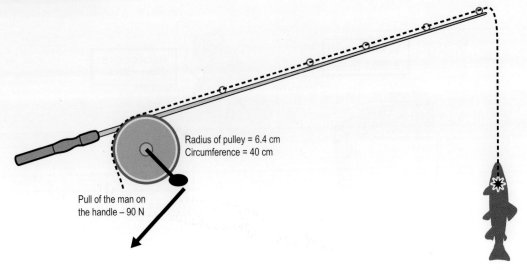

Radius of pulley = 6.4 cm
Circumference = 40 cm

Pull of the man on
the handle – 90 N

Figure 5.4 • Fishing rod.

the fish into shore. He pulls on the handle with 90 N; the handle is 0.064 m from the centre of the reel. The circumference of the reel is 40 cm. The man turns the reel three times to lift the fish. How much work does he perform? (see Fig. 5.4).

Answers for both questions are in Appendix 5.

Direction of work

As we have said work is a scalar quantity because part of its calculation—distance (which could be linear or angular)—is a scalar. This means we do not need to state a direction; however, work can be positive or negative. If the applied force is in the same direction as the resulting movement of the body, as in throwing a baseball, then the work is positive. If, however, the force is applied against the motion (as in catching a baseball) then the work is negative.

In the body, muscles perform positive work when the pulling force they apply to a bone(s) causes joint movement in the same direction as the muscle pull; e.g. if you straighten your leg while you are sitting there, the quadriceps shorten to pull on your lower leg (via the patella) which obligingly rotates round (straightens). This is positive work or could be described as a concentric contraction (see pp. 9-10 for further details). The muscle shortens and the bone moves in the same direction.

Negative work is performed when the bone(s) move in the opposite direction of the muscle pull; e.g. with your leg straightened out in front of you, lower it down slowly to the ground. The knee is flexing; however, the quadriceps are working reasonably hard to oppose this motion (or at least control it), which means that the muscle must lengthen as it continues to pull on the bone. This type of muscle activity is negative work or could also be described as an eccentric contraction.

So work is performed when a force (like a muscle pull) changes a body's (or body segment) position. It could be positive or negative.

Vertical jumping provides a good illustration of muscle work. On the way up the muscles that extend the hips, knees and ankles provide a huge amount of positive work (depending on the size of person and how high they want to jump); on landing this reverses as the same muscles perform a huge amount (similar to the amount of work on the way up) of negative work: the hips, knees and ankles flex while the extensors create tension to slow down the rate of flexion.

CD-ROM activity 5.1: Jumping

Using machines to do work

The genius of man has been in the development of machines to help them perform work, whether this is a plough to push soil aside or a can opener to ... well you know what that does! They have the same purpose: to make it easier to perform work on another body. A machine is simply a device that can help you do work. You put work in (e.g. muscle work) and you get work out (e.g. lifting a box).

The lever is the simplest machine used by man. So simple in fact that it is used by other primates as well. You might have seen pictures of monkeys using sticks to lift up boulders so they can get at the tasty ants. We are going to talk about levers in the following section as it builds on our understanding of moments and work and because it provides further insight into the way the musculoskeletal system works. You could say our skeletal system is a simple system of levers, but that would diminish the human body.

A lever consists of four components: a rigid beam, a pivot (or fulcrum), effort and load; see Figure 5.5.

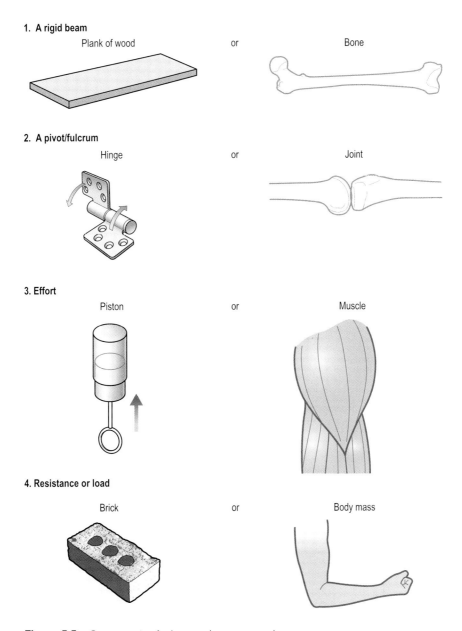

1. A rigid beam

Plank of wood   or   Bone

2. A pivot/fulcrum

Hinge   or   Joint

3. Effort

Piston   or   Muscle

4. Resistance or load

Brick   or   Body mass

Figure 5.5 • Components of a lever and some examples.

The main purpose behind the design of a lever is that it provides something called mechanical advantage over the object you are trying to move, be it a child on a seesaw or the door of a safe.

Mechanical advantage is simply the ratio of load to effort. Consider a burglar trying to prise open a safe. The lock on the safe is held by a steel bolt which is capable of resisting forces of 2000 N; it is located 0.1 m from the hinge so can resist turning forces of 200 Nm (2000 × 0.1 m). A person is unlikely to generate this type of force; however, by using the principle of moments a lever (in this case a crow bar) inserted into the lock can. If a robber applies a force of 133 N at a point 1.5 m along the lever (from the pivot point), he can generate the necessary 200 Nm required to bust the lock and steal the jewels: (see Fig. 5.6)

Applied force (133 N) × perpendicular distance from fulcrum (1.5 m) = 200 Nm

So, the load that must be overcome is 2000 N and effort (push) is 133 N, which means the advantage is 15 times (the same as the perpendicular distance). The mechanical advantage comes from the ability to locate the effort force further away from the pivot than the load. The use of the lever makes the job 15 times easier.

Let's say a 20-kg load of wood is sitting in a wheelbarrow and has to be moved. The mass of the wood generates a downward force of 20 kg (mass) × 9.81 (acceleration due to gravity) = 196.2 N. This force is applied 0.5 m behind the fulcrum (wheel axis). Therefore the wood creates a turning force (moment) of 98 Nm (196.2 N × 0.5 m); see Figure 5.7. To lift the load therefore requires a force to match or exceed this.

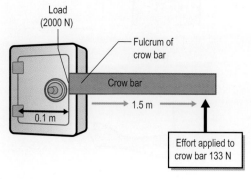

Figure 5.6 • Using a lever to open a safe.

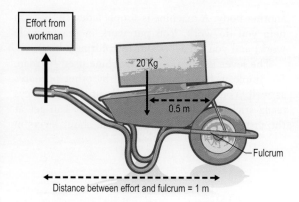

Figure 5.7 • A wheelbarrow.

The force the workman applies to lift the wheelbarrow level is located 1 m from the fulcrum (i.e. double the distance that the load of wood is from the axis), which means to create the 98 Nm (rotational force of wood) only requires a force of 98 N (half of the force of the wood). Or to put it another way:

98 N (workman's force) × 1 m (distance to fulcrum) = 196.2 (force of wood pile) × 0.5 (distance to fulcrum)

Therefore the mechanical advantage is 196.2/98 = 2.
Try the next question yourself:

Question 4

A man is holding a 2-kg tin of chopped tomatoes in his hand. The combined mass of the tomatoes and his forearm is 6 kg, which produces a force of 6 × 9.81 = 58.9 N. This force is located approximately 40 cm from the elbow. The combination of force and distance from joint creates an extension moment (rotational force trying to straighten the elbow) 58.9 N × 0.4 = 23.5 Nm. The elbow flexors (muscles that bend the elbow) apply their opposing rotational force (flexor moment) at a closer distance, i.e. 5 cm. This means to hold the tomatoes the elbow flexors must produce a force of ___? Answer is in Appendix 5 (see Fig. 5.8).

Categories of levers

🔘 CD-ROM activity 5.2

Right, so now we know that levers are simple machines and that they help you perform work.

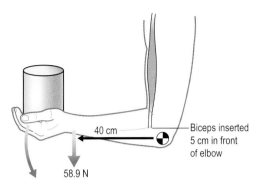

Figure 5.8 • How much force do the elbow flexors have to produce to hold the tin of tomatoes?

The more distance from the pivot you can place your effort (compared to the load), the greater the mechanical advantage. You may have noticed from the questions that levers are arranged in different ways that alter their mechanical advantage. In fact there are three arrangements of lever.

The first type, type 1, is the classic seesaw (or tee-ter-totter if you live in the USA (Fig. 5.9)) arrangement where the effort and load are located on either side of the pivot. Mechanical advantage is then dependent on how far away each is from the pivot.

There are not many examples of this type of lever in the human body; perhaps the most obvious is when you nod your head. The neck is the pivot for this movement, the pull of the neck extensors is the effort and the load is the mass of the head (it has more mass towards the front) (Fig. 5.10).

The second type of lever is where both the effort and load/resistance are located on the same

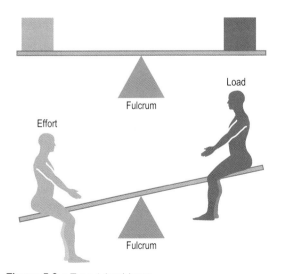

Figure 5.9 • Type 1 (one) lever.

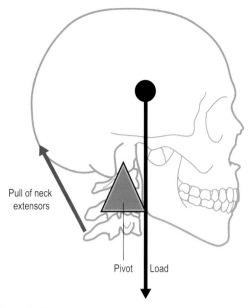

Figure 5.10 • Nodding as an example of a type 1 lever.

side (see Fig. 5.11). An everyday example of this is the wheel barrow (see Fig. 5.7). Can you think of any other examples?

Because of the way a type 2 lever is arranged the effort force will always be further away from the pivot than the load, so it will always be at a mechanical advantage. Again there are few examples of this lever arrangement in the human body. Textbooks typically refer to the movement of going up onto the balls of your feet.

The tables are turned for the type 3 lever. The effort and load are still located on the same side but this time the load is furthest away from the fulcrum (see Fig. 5.12).

This is a little like a baseball player striking a ball. Think about the ball as the load and hands as the effort and, this may vary but let's think of the pivot as the shoulder, i.e. a third class lever.

This lever arrangement is very common in the human body (see Fig. 5.13 and try Practical Activity 5.1).

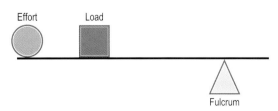

Figure 5.11 • Type 2 (two) lever.

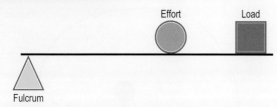

Figure 5.12 • Type 3 (three) lever.

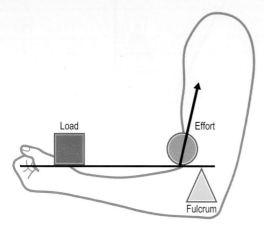

Figure 5.13 • Elbow flexion as an example of type 3 lever.

Consider the following items and state which type of lever they are (clue: just identify the fulcrum, effort and load; then it should be obvious):

1. Crane

2. Scissors

3. Bottle opener

4. Drawbridge of a castle

Then try Practical Activity 5.2

CD-ROM activity 5.3

Practical Activity Box 5.1

Roll your sleeve up and look at your arm. Find the centre of the elbow from the side (the fulcrum). Now find the effort. This could be the biceps at the front or triceps (elbow extensors) at the back of the elbow. Now identify where the load is. This is the mass of the forearm, which is around 2–4 kg and is located at the CoM (about a third of the way between the elbow and the tip of the fingers. When you extend your arm, for example reaching out for a pencil, what type of lever arrangement is the triceps working in? Answer is in Appendix 5.

Practical Activity Box 5.2

Place the levers below in order of their mechanical advantage (easiest for the effort) (clue: you may need a ruler).

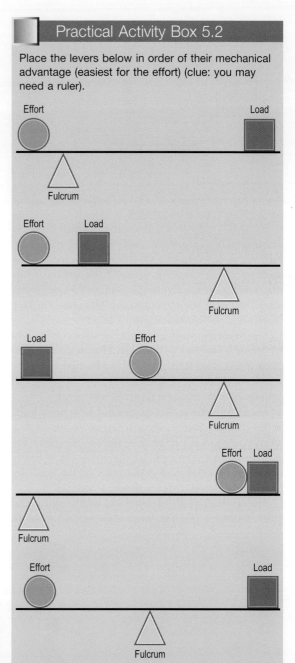

Figure 5.14 • Practical activity 5.2; placing levers in order of mechanical advantage.

Velocity ratio

Given what we have just said about mechanical advantage for the type 3 levers and how common this arrangement is within the human body, an obvious question might be why have we evolved what appears to be an inefficient system?

The reason is something called velocity ratio. This is the ratio of the **distance moved by the effort** (at the point of application) and the **distance moved by the load**.

Let's take the example of opening a door: we have used mechanical advantage in putting the point of application of our pull furthest away from the pivot. This does mean that we must pull the door handle a greater angular distance than if we pulled next to the hinge. If we did apply our pull close to the hinge, it would certainly be harder in terms of force, but you wouldn't need to pull as far. Muscles are inserted close to joint centres for this reason; they don't have to shorten as much (so you can do it faster) to create the same change in angle as if they were placed far away.

To illustrate this let's get back to the lifting a weight example. By shortening the biceps muscle by a few centimetres the elbow can move through 30°. If the muscle was inserted further along the bone towards the load, its mechanical advantage would be increased but it would have to move through a larger distance with the consequential reduction in velocity (see Fig. 5.15). We need to be able to execute movements relatively quickly; therefore muscles are inserted in this manner. Speed over efficiency is often what we need.

More advanced machines

Levers are an example of a machine that can help you perform work. During the industrial revolution, simple lever machines were replaced with more

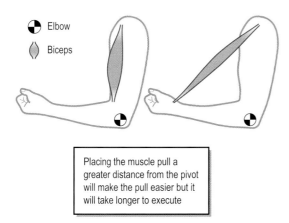

Elbow

Biceps

Placing the muscle pull a greater distance from the pivot will make the pull easier but it will take longer to execute

Figure 5.15 • Velocity versus mechanical efficiency.

sophisticated machines capable of doing heavier and faster work (although not always more efficiently), particularly in trades that required the movement of large loads e.g. mining, shipping and farming. Many of these machines were first invented by the ancient Greeks. Some of these machines are used in sport and rehabilitation, although sometimes their objective is not to make the task easier but harder!

Pulleys

The pulley is a machine that consists of a wheel with a free (minimal friction) moving axle about which the wheel spins. The wheel has a groove around its circumference and a rope which fits into the groove. It works because the rope grips the wheel and causes it to turn. It has a long nautical history where it is called a block and tackle. The basic pulley (type 1) is a simple arrangement of a wheel fixed to a stable surface (e.g. floor or wall), see Figure 5.16. A rope is passed through the groove; at one end of the rope is the load/weight and at the other end is the effort.

The purpose of a simple pulley is that it changes the direction of the force. This is particularly useful if you want to take advantage of gravity to lift an object up rather than pushing it up (see Fig. 5.16B). There is no mechanical advantage; the force you pull with is translated directly to the force that pulls the load up. Well, this is theoretically the case; however, some of the force you apply is opposed by friction (see previous chapter for details on friction, p. 59) in the movement of the pulley wheel. The sliding friction of the rope through the groove will also produce heat, which is not terribly useful and something that must be controlled or it could lead to disastrous results.

Historically this simple setup served a range of different jobs; however, things became more interesting when pulleys became moveable (not solidly fixed to a stone or tree but able to move via the rope. These are sometimes referred to as type 2 pulleys and are generally credited to Archimedes (see Further Information Box 5.3). The reason for the excitement is that this arrangement requires much less effort; the trade-off is that more rope must be pulled to gain the same elevation (a bit like when we moved the biceps along the arm: less effort but more muscle must be used; Fig. 5.15).

Simple pulley

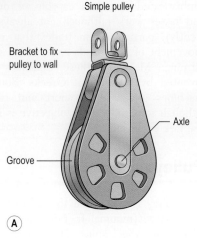

Bracket to fix pulley to wall

Axle

Groove

A

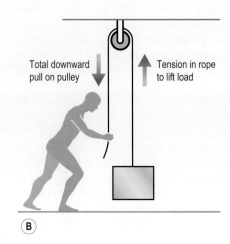

Total downward pull on pulley

Tension in rope to lift load

B

Figure 5.16 • Type 1 (simple) pulley.

The type 2 pulley is designed so that the pulley itself can move (not rigidly attached to the wall like a type 1; Fig. 5.16): when the person pulls the rope the pulley moves up. Now in this situation the force to lift the object is halved; however, the distance you have to pull the rope doubles. So the work (force × distance) remains the same but each pull is easier (useful for heavy loads). Now you might find this arrangement a little awkward but you can always add another pulley to change the direction.

Now if there are two (moveable) pulleys we can reduce the force required even further but at the same time the distance the load moves for each pull will reduce. So more pulls but each one is easier (Fig. 5.17).

The simple type 1 pulley is widely used in rehabilitation. This can be used to assist a movement, e.g. shoulder flexion by the pull of a stronger limb, e.g. opposite shoulder extension. It can also provide a means of resisting a movement with the opposite limb creating a greater load (through active resistance) for the exercising arm.

Pulleys in the human body

The principle behind the simple pulley has not gone unnoticed by nature. While there are no true replicas of pulleys in the body there are plenty of examples of a change in the direction of a muscle pull helped by grooves in bones. Consider the action of the quadriceps muscle as it (via the patella) glides over the femoral groove (just like the groove in the wheel of a pulley) so that it can pull on the tibial condyle. This arrangement also increases the perpendicular distance between the knee joint centre and muscle pull, creating a larger moment for the quadriceps (see Fig. 5.18).

A similar example can be seen in the long flexors of the fingers: the pull of the muscle tendon is redirected by the tendinous straps attached to the bones so that angular motion across several joints is created by the pull of one tendon. This anatomical feature is often described as a pulley although it is not a true pulley; see Figure 5.19A. Given our

Type 2 pulley:
effort halved, distance doubled

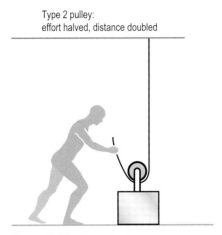

Figure 5.17 • Type 2 pulley.

Two type 2 pulleys:
effort quartered

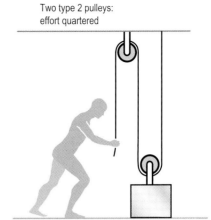

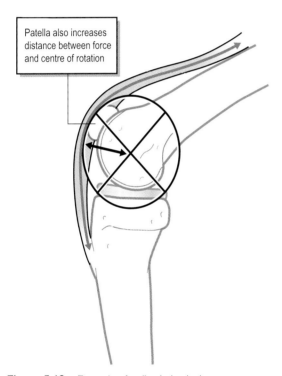

Patella also increases
distance between force
and centre of rotation

Figure 5.18 • Example of pulley in body, knee.

complicated shape it is not really surprising that we have so many changes in muscle direction. Perhaps the closest thing to a pulley in the human body is the action of peroneus longus, which is a muscle positioned on the outside of the lower leg that rotates the foot outwards. The pull of this muscle is redirected by one of the bones in the foot (cuboid) to transfer its pull from the lateral to medial side of the foot (see Fig. 5.19B). The pull

causes the foot to rotate (like the spinning pulley) about an axis centred on the subtalar joint (under the ankle joint).

The power of work

When we talk about how muscles work, power is an important factor. Although often used synonymously with strength, **power** is actually the rate (or how quickly) the work (force × distance) is being done so you need to consider time. Power is calculated as the work done divided by the time taken. The units are joules per second or, more simply, watts (W), after the Scottish inventor of the steam engine, James Watts, the real power behind the Industrial Revolution and the man who coined the term *horsepower*.

Let's say you want to lift a box and you have sensibly set up a pulley to do this. The box weighs 20 kg so you must pull with a force exceeding 200 N (mass of 20 kg × acceleration of gravity which as you recall has a value of 9.81). So you pull down with a force 250 N and the box moves vertically by 35 cm (0.35 m) (see Fig. 5.20); this means the work you perform is 250 N × 0.35 m = 87.5 J. If it takes you 5 seconds to perform this elevation, the power you have expended is 17.5 (87.5/5) J/s or simply 17.5 W.

So what about muscle power? Just like machines the power of a muscle is its ability to generate work rapidly. You should make the distinction between muscle strength, which is simply the ability of the muscle to generate work (this is also called tension because muscles always pull; you could also think of it as strength), and muscle power, which is how rapidly it can perform work, or generate tension.

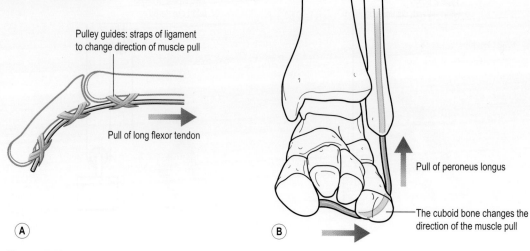

Figure 5.19 • Examples of pulley in body: (A) Finger flexion, (B) Peroneus longus and cuboid.

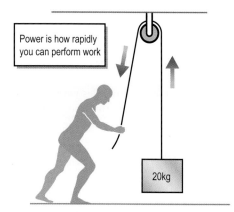

Figure 5.20 • Power during a lift.

Let's get back to the standing up from a chair movement. If you recall (Fig. 5.3) we calculated that during the sit-to-stand movement the quadriceps muscle group created a turning force of 200 Nm which moved the thigh (and therefore the rest of the body) through an arc of 30 cm (an angle of 0.75 rad (0.3m/0.4m) or 43°). This means that 150 J of work (200 Nm × 0.75 rad) was performed by the quadriceps group of muscles. So what about power?

The average time (based on literature) to perform the extension phase of the sit-to-stand movement (thighs horizontal to thighs vertical) is 0.5 s. Power, as you now know, is work divided by time; therefore at this speed the quadriceps group would perform:

150 J/0.5 s = 300 W of power

Interestingly muscle power has been reported to decrease proportionally more than strength with ageing. Amongst other things this has manifested in a slower standing up time from sitting; values of 2–3 seconds have been reported. Let's say an older person takes 2.5 s to straighten up; this would mean (if we assume the same values of mass and distance) a power value of

150/2.5 = 60 W

which is a reduction of 80%!

It has been suggested that, for a frail older person, standing up from a chair is as difficult as a maximum vertical jump (jumping as high as you can from a standing position) is for a young person. Let's look at the power required to perform a vertical jump.

Let's say an average person (mass 75 kg) performs a maximal standing jump. They squat down and apply a pushing force to the ground that exceeds their body weight and therefore the body accelerates, vertically lifting off the ground. If we estimate the value of this force is around 2.5 × body weight (to take into account the additional force required to accelerate the body up off the ground), so 75 × gravity (9.81) × 2.5 = 1840 N. Since this lifts the body by 40 cm then the work done is 1840 × 0.4 = 736 J. This work is carried out rapidly (let's say 0.4 s), which means the power is 736 divided by 0.4 = 1840 W.

This is quite a difference from the 60 W expended (theoretically) by an older slow person getting out of a chair. The reason it is suggested to be similar to a vertical jump is that this 60 W represents a similar proportion of the available muscle power in an old person as 1840 does in a younger fit person performing a vertical jump, i.e. both near maximum!

 CD-ROM activity 5.4

Efficiency

We have already discussed **efficiency** a little but it is worth spending a little more time on it because it is a popular theme in human movement studies. By understanding how much energy is lost in the performance of a task, a greater insight into the way the body moves can be gained. In Chapter 9 we will discuss the ways in which the human body acts to maximize efficiency; suffice to say we are naturally parsimonious when it comes to movement.

In mechanical terms efficiency is calculated as the ratio between the work put in (input) and the work done (output). You will come across the term in many areas of life. When buying a car you may be interested in how many miles it does to the gallon: how much energy (in this case the chemical energy created by the combustion of petrol) do you have to input to get the output (displacement of the car—miles). It's quite a challenge to calculate all the ways in which efficiency can be lost; however, it is fairly straightforward to measure efficiency. It is simply the output divided by the input. This is then expressed as a percentage. Let's get back to our comfort zone when we talk about machines, the seesaw (see Fig. 5.21).

We can work out the work required to lift the child. The child weighs 25 kg (so the force of the child is $25 \times 9.81 = 245$ N) and (provided the seesaw is rigid) moves vertically by 0.5 m; therefore the work output is 122.5 J. Let's say the amount of work put in was 125 J (250 N $\times$ 0.5 m); 5 N more was required so the ratio is

$$\frac{122.5 \text{ (work output)}}{125 \text{ (work input)}} = 0.98 \text{ or } 98\%$$

A value of almost 100% means that practically all the effort put in was converted to work lifting the child. This would be a very efficient machine. But what about the 2%? The process of performing work inevitably means some energy will be converted to another form of energy. For example overcoming friction as well as some air resistance will have resulted in some of the input energy being transferred from accomplishing the movement task.

No system is truly perfect in terms of efficiency. In real life, as a general rule, the simpler the machine the more efficient it is. The type of engine in a traditional motorcar, along with the vast number of moving parts, lowers its efficiency to around 40%, so more than half the energy created from the petrol is lost to heat. This is, however, an advance on the old-fashioned steam engines which only used 15% of the consumed energy for work. In a simple bicycle the efficiency (see Further Information Box 5.4) is almost ideal with values around 95–99%! Although the addition of gears to the

 Further Information Box 5.4

The efficiency of the bicycle

Simple pulleys and gears lie at the heart of the most popular invention of the human race—the bicycle.[1] The reason for its popularity is that it satisfies all the basic requirements of a machine: easy to use (well perhaps not for your average 3-year-old), inexpensive, easy to repair and most importantly reduces the amount of work required. In fact the bicycle has been demonstrated to be the most efficient mode of road transport in terms of the ratio between work in and work out.

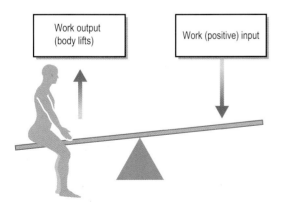

Figure 5.21 ● Example of efficiency; lifting a child on a seesaw.

[1]According to a recent poll carried out in the UK by the British Broadcasting Corporation (BBC), 59% voted for the common bicycle, compared to 4% for the Internet and 5% for the radio.

modern bike has reduced this efficiency a little it represents an efficient means of transport.

The efficiency of humans has been studied from movement and dietary perspectives. After all if we know how much energy an activity costs we can estimate how much energy we need (in terms of food) and perhaps more importantly how much we don't need.

The problem lies in calculating a human's energy expenditure. The accepted best way is to use a physiological technique based on the amount of oxygen you use up (consume) while carrying out the activity. The gases you breathe out are analysed (this means wearing a mask) and the percentage of CO_2 is calculated and compared with normal percentage in air. This tells us how much O_2 was used

and therefore the amount of energy (once you have subtracted the amount used when resting).

We will return to the issue of energy and efficiency in Chapter 9 when we talk about functional movements and the clever anatomical designs that make us more efficient.

What you need to remember from that bit

Mechanical **work** is the application of force to move a body. Levers are simple tools consisting of a rigid beam (bone), fulcrum (joint), effort (muscle) and load (body weight/external load) to help us do work. There are three types of lever. The first type

---

Further Information Box 5.5

Perpetual motion machines

For many years the Holy Grail in the design of machines was the perpetual motion machine. The idea that captured the imagination of many inventors was the possibility of a machine that could run without an energy source: once started it would continue to move (perform work) forever. Can you imagine how famous you would be in today's energy-stricken world if you came up with a machine like that!

As we have said a machine performs work, e.g. lifting a heavy load. To do this a machine needs energy which is used in two ways: (1) to move the object (kinetic energy being used) and (2) frictional generation of other energy forms (typically heat; thermal energy). If you add the heat energy and kinetic energy together the total amount expended will equal the energy put in. In other words all the energy can, theoretically, be accounted for, even if only a portion is used for the actual work.

The fact that these machines are actually impossible because they contravene the basic laws of physics, energy input must equal energy output, and there must be some, even miniscule loss of energy from the system, has not deterred some intrepid inventors.

Of course, the so-called, perpetual motion machines that do exist only give the appearance of work being done without any obvious input of energy. However, these machines do rely on energy sources. The bobbing of the drinking bird toy is caused by a process of pressure changes instigated by evaporation and condensation, which are caused by the temperature of

the room; i.e. it is the heat energy that keeps this amusing toy moving—it wouldn't work in a cold room.

Why not conduct an Internet search for perpetual motion machines and see if you can work out where the energy comes from.

CD-ROM activity 5.5

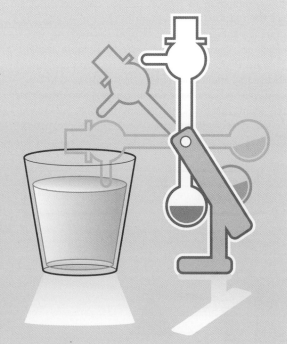

Figure 5.22 • A perpetual motion machine.

places the effort and load on either side of a fulcrum (like a seesaw), the second type sees the effort and load on same side of the fulcrum with the effort furthest away (effort has the advantage), and the third type also has the effort and load on the same side, but this time the load is furthest away (load has mechanical advantage).

Power is the rate of doing work (work divided by time) and measured in watts. The power of muscle activity is different from strength and appears to reduce more with age than strength alone.

That's us all done with forces!

Well, not really but in the next couple of chapters we are going to look at how tissue behaves when forces are applied to them but before we do that it is worth checking your understanding of force and movement (in an applied way). This isn't a test but if you can work out the answers then you should consider yourself well on the way to biomechanical enlightenment.

Practical problems on force and human movement

Fold a single sock up into a smallish square and place it inside one of your shoes so that it will be under your heel when you put the shoe on. What you have done is not too dissimilar (in a Heath Robinson kind of way) to a method used by podiatrists and physiotherapists to reduce strain on an injured Achilles tendon (heel chord).

Now stand up and feel the difference between your feet. You should feel a change in how your pressure is distributed at your feet. The centre of pressure (where the ground reaction force is, on average, located) should have shifted forwards a little on the sock side, perhaps under the ball of your foot but of course this will depend on the thickness of the sock you used!

Can you feel any difference at your ankle, knee, hip, back?

Have a think about how the relationship between your joints and the ground reaction force has changed now that it is being applied further forwards on your foot.

Compare both sides. Are the same muscles working to the same extent?

For further information on this problem why not look up the experimental study by Reinschmidt and Nigg from 1994.

There are some comments on this problem in Appendix 5.

Now that you are standing up let's move onto a walking problem. Take the sock out of your shoe and stand somewhere that you will be able to walk for a few minutes, e.g. corridor, pavement, and make sure the area is clear. Now walk forwards for a few minutes and remind yourself what kind of moments are being created in the lower limb and where they are being created. If you need a wee reminder then try the CD-ROM activity 5.6.

CD-ROM activity 5.6

Now stop and walk backwards. Have a think about how the forces have changed. The magnitude of the force is likely to be the same, assuming you have not lost mass in the past 5 minutes and you are walking at the same speed as you did in forward walking.

The first point of contact is now the forefoot. How does this change the moments about your ankle and how does this affect muscle activity?

The foot is then gently lowered backwards, but which muscle group controls this movement? Remember when walking forwards that the dorsiflexors (eccentrically) controlled the plantarflexion.

Sometimes to understand a movement problem it is worth adopting the posture, feeling where the pressure is and how the muscles are working. So for the next problem let's try that. Stand up and bend your trunk forwards a little. Now take note of any changes in the centre of pressure at your feet. How are your muscles working compared to when you were standing straight? Think about how your CoM has moved and how this has altered the moments about your lower limbs. This time try to focus on your knee. How have the forces changed at this joint when you are bent forward?

Why do you think some people put themselves into this posture when they stand and walk? What possible advantage does it give them in terms of muscle work or altered pressure? Why do you think cyclists adopt this bent posture when they are struggling up hills, crouched over their handlebars?

OK let's try another movement problem: You sit down on a sofa in your friend's house and their very friendly dog comes along and lies under your knees so that your feet are pushed forwards from the sofa. When you come to stand up you find it pretty difficult to do and not because you have consumed too many beers. Can you explain why this has happened? Think about where your mass is and where you are applying the force.

Finally here is another walking problem: Walking along you come upon a sign that reads 'Careful. Floor is slippery. Danger of falling.'

Being a careful person you take heed of this warning. Explain why a slippery floor presents a greater risk of falling and then describe how you would adjust your walking pattern to minimize your risk of falling.

Clue: First try it out (but don't actually use a slippery floor, just pretend) and then think about the direction of the forces. Remember that you are applying forces to the ground through your lower limb so the angle it makes with the ground will be important.

The answers to these problems are given in Appendix 5.

Chapter **Six**

6

Stress and Strain

What you will learn about in this chapter
1. The types of stress;
2. The types of strain;
3. The relationship between stress and strain (stiffness and elasticity); and
4. How materials can flow with time.

Words you will come across
Stress, strain, elasticity, plasticity, stiffness, viscosity, thixotropy.

Up to this point, when we talked about the action of force on bodies, we considered the body to be rigid. It didn't stretch or get squashed when the force was applied. Of course, this is not the case with the human body. We have many soft bits that squash and stretch when they are pushed and pulled. The forces that squash and squeeze tissues such as our skin, bone or tendon might be a sudden single impact from a fall or repeated applications during a cyclical activity like running or using a keyboard. Understanding how tissues cope with these different types of force application is fundamental to understanding injury and repair. In this chapter you will be introduced to the area of material science. Chapter 7 will talk more specifically about the tissues of the human body, i.e. tissue mechanics.

The body is a wonderful piece of engineering. Aeons of natural selection have resulted in the human body being constructed from a range of materials designed for specific functions; e.g. bone provides

a rigid beam for muscles to create moments whereas skin provides a stretchable, protective, waterproof barrier. Imagine if these characteristics were swapped? By preventing natural expansion after a large dinner, rigid skin would make Christmas afternoon quite uncomfortable while stretchy bone would pose quite a few problems for those of us hoping to actually get out of bed.

Understanding how materials in general behave when forces are applied to them is a good starting place for this chapter. This will allow me to introduce some key principles before we move on to understanding how these principles apply to human tissues.

Definitions

Engineers have long been interested in how materials cope with force. If you are building a bridge you need to know that the materials you use can endure the repetitive compressing loads from cars and lorries as well as high winds which will push and pull the bridge at different speeds and in multiple directions. The same could be said for clothes designers; they need to know just how far the elastic in your pants can stretch and how often, before they fail.

So, it should be no surprise that the mechanical properties of most materials have been scientifically tested. Material science has its own principles and terminology which can be applied just as appropriately to the human body as they are to concrete pillars in bridges or the elastic in your pants. After all, just like engineers we need to know why and how the supportive structures of the body, e.g. bones and mucles, fail and perhaps more importantly how to repair them. Let's start this understanding with a couple of important terms.

Stress

When speaking about materials, **stress** or **load** is the force applied to a material per unit area, i.e. force divided by area, which means the units are Nm^{-2}. The observant amongst you will have noticed this is the same as pressure. Although the terms stress, pressure and load could be considered synonymous, in this context, for clarity we will just use the term stress.

Stress can be applied to a material in different directions.

Compressive stress

Compressive stress is a pushing stress. It means that it is pushing vertically down onto the surface of the body so that it is at right angles to it, i.e. perpendicular (Fig. 6.1). For example if you put a balloon between your hands and squeezed it or when you sit on top of an overfull suitcase to try to close it.

Many structures in the body experience compressive stress. Think of the bones in your leg being squashed by the weight of your body while you are standing, or if you are sitting, consider the weight of your head, arms and trunk squashing the skin of your buttocks. Gravity certainly causes a lot of compression. Perhaps the most easily illustrated example of compressive stress is in the spine where the vertebral bodies and intervertebral discs must endure a long day of being squashed from the mass of your head, arms and trunk, in sitting and standing (see Fig. 6.2).

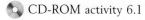 CD-ROM activity 6.1

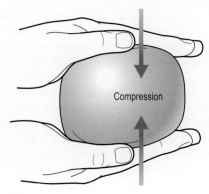

Figure 6.1 • Compressive force.

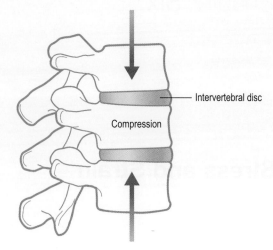

Figure 6.2 • Compression force on a vertebral body.

Tensile stress

Tensile stress is a pulling stress. Like compressive stress it is also applied perpendicularly to the surface of the body but this time it is directed away from the body, for example if you pulled a spring open or stretched a balloon or elastic band (see Fig. 6.3).

When you think about it, lots of the bits in our body are subjected to pulling stress. The tendons

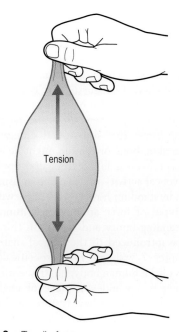

Figure 6.3 • Tensile force.

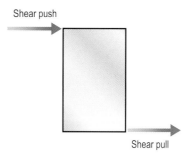

Figure 6.5 • Shear stress.

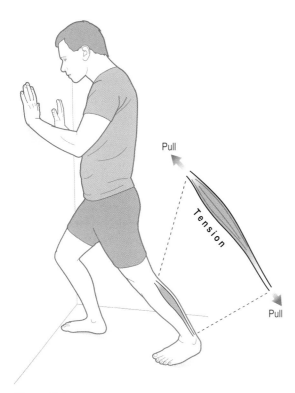

Figure 6.4 • Tensile force on a muscle.

endure tensile stress with every muscle contraction. This even occurs when the body part is moved passively, like a passive stretch (see Fig. 6.4) from a sports therapist. Next time you walk home from the supermarket holding bags of shopping in both hands, you will now know that the uncomfortable feeling in your shoulders is due to the tensile stress produced by the downward pull of the bags.

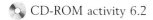 CD-ROM activity 6.2

Shear stress

Shear stress is a little more difficult to explain. It can be either a push or a pull but it is applied **horizontally** to a specified plane of a body. So, it acts parallel to a given surface rather than perpendicular to it as in the case of tensile and compressive (see Fig. 6.5). Try Practical Activity 6.1. It might help you to understand what I am trying to explain.

Shear stress is experienced by lots of different body structures, depending on what you are doing. For example think of yourself just now sitting on a chair. If you slide down the chair a little the skin

Practical Activity Box 6.1

Applying shear stress causes individual layers of a material within the body to slide over each other (even if this is microscopically). Get a large book. A deck of cards would also work (although not as well) if gambling, not reading, is your preference.

Lie the book on a roughish surface (so it won't slide) and press along the top of the front cover as indicated in Figure 6.6. If you do it correctly you should see the pages of the book slide on top of each other, stopped eventually by the binding. Be careful not to push too far back because you will damage the binding.

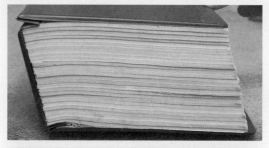

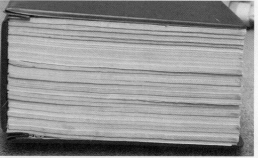

Figure 6.6 • Shear stress, practical activity 6.1.

on your back (if you were resting on a backrest) and buttocks will experience shear stress, top surface being stretched, and the layers underneath sliding on each other, just like the book (see Fig. 6.6). If friction is minimal and the layers are allowed to slide, then fine. If, however, there is friction between the layers there is the possibility they can become crumpled, causing damage and loss of function.

Basically if one body slides across the surface of another then shear stress will result. The parts of the body that experiences this most often and with high forces are the joint surfaces. The articular cartilage that lines the joint surfaces is designed specifically to cope with shear stress. They try to cope with shear stress by reducing the friction between the layers as they slide over each other; this reduces any crumpling effect (more on this in Chapter 7).

Most joints don't function as a simple hinge joint (Fig. 6.7). There are additional rotations (spin) as well as translation (slipping), forward/backward and side to side (Fig. 6.8). These movements are important to the mobility of the joint but create **shear forces** on the joint surface.

Bending stress

Bending stress is a mixture of compressive and tensile. Imagine sitting on a beam of wood balanced between two chairs (not sure when you would do this but try to imagine). You would expect the beam to bend a little in the middle (depending on its flexibility and your mass) (see Fig. 6.9). What's happening in the beam is that the top layers of wood are being pushed together—compression—while the bottom layers are pulled apart—tension. This difference means that the layers of the material must slide on each other; i.e. shear stress must also exist in bending.

Bending forces are a frequent occurrence for bones in the body. Consider the head of the femur when loaded (see Fig. 6.10).

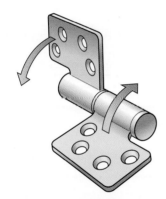

Figure 6.7 • Hinge.

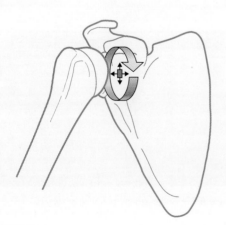

Figure 6.8 • Translation and pin of humerus in shoulder.

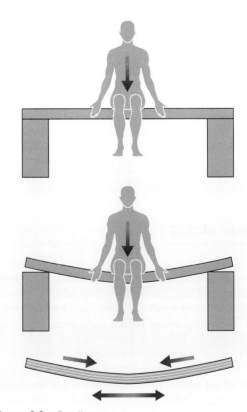

Figure 6.9 • Bending stress.

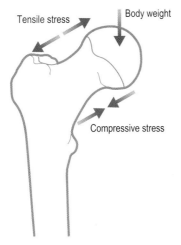

Figure 6.10 • Stresses on head of femur.

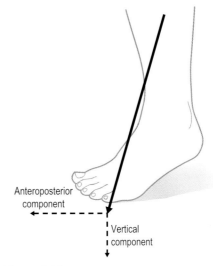

Figure 6.12 • Forces at the metatarsal heads when jogging.

Torsional stress or rotational stress

You could think of torsional stress like the twisting force you might use to break off a bit of soft candy or a chunk of French bread. This twisting motion actually results in shear stresses at different points on the body and in different directions (see Fig. 6.11).

Let's see if you can remember all that with a quick test. Identify the type of stress in the following situations.

(A) The foot while jogging

When your foot strikes the ground while you are out jogging it is typically the metatarsal heads (ball of feet) that touch first (although this does depend on how fast you run) (see Fig. 6.12). So what kind of stress do you think the tissue (skin, bursa, tendons and fatty pads) under the metatarsal heads experiences at foot strike?

As the foot strikes the ground there will be large forces generated as the momentum of the body is rapidly reduced. This braking force will be felt in

different directions (vertical, side to side and forwards and back) because the momentum of the body exists in these directions. The vertical and anteroposterior direction are shown in Figure 6.12.

- What kind of stress does the anteroposterior horizontal component cause at the metatarsal heads?
  - ○ Bending
  - ○ Torsional
  - ○ Shear
  - ○ Compressive
- What kind of stress does the vertical component cause at the metatarsal heads?
  - ○ Bending
  - ○ Torsional
  - ○ Shear
  - ○ Compressive
- What could happen with repetitive application of these stresses?

(B) A blow to the back of the knee

Imagine you are attending a game of soccer. You see a particularly bad tackle with one player kicking the back of the knee of another player causing his tibia to slide forward on the femur.

- What type of stress is experienced by the articular surface from the movement of the tibia?
- What type of stress does the anterior cruciate experience? The anterior cruciate is a strong ligament orientated to prevent the tibia sliding forward, as indicated in Figure 6.13.

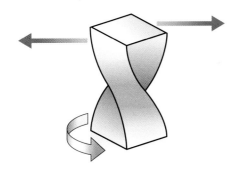

Figure 6.11 • Torsional stress.

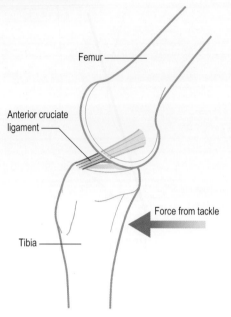

Femur

Anterior cruciate ligament

Force from tackle

Tibia

Figure 6.13 • The anterior cruciate under stress.

- What do you think could happen to the anterior cruciate with this kind of stress? Answers in Appendix 6.

OK, we have talked about different kinds of stress including eating burgers (see Practical Activity 6.2); now let's consider the effects of stress.

Strain

Strain is another word used by many professionals—e.g. a medical doctor might say 'You have strained your ankle ligament'—as well as in everyday language—'The last couple of weeks have been a real strain.' In material science, it specifically relates to the change in shape of a body. This could be lengthening, which is positive strain, or compression, which is negative strain. It is calculated by dividing the change in dimension, e.g. length, by the original dimension. So, basically strain is the relative change in shape of a body under stress.

For example, let's say you have an elastic band 12 cm long when unstretched (lying on the table in front of you). You pick it up and stretch it between your hands (tensile stress) and of course it increases in size, let's say to 17 cm, which means it changed by 5 cm (17 cm – 12 cm). The strain then would be 5 (change in length)/12 (original length) = 0.4167, which we convert to a percentage, so the strain would be 41.67%.

This strain, caused by tension, is called tensile strain, as there was an increase in length. An important part of this process is the change in energy state of the elastic band. Now that you have stretched it, it has potential energy due to its elasticity. If you let go it would ping back. Every child knows this as they

Practical Activity Box 6.2

When you next have a big burger, or any big sandwich really, and bite down on it, think about the stress you are applying: compression at the front where you are biting and tension at the back where the burger opens up. This will probably result in the ketchup or other content falling onto the table or more annoyingly onto your lap. This has occurred due to the difference in pressure between the front and back of the burger. We will look more at movement within the body due to pressure differences, in Chapter 8.

Does this hamburger analogy bring to mind any part of the body?

The intervertebral discs experience much the same pattern of stress application, but in this instance it won't be the ketchup that moves: it's the centre of the vertebral disc, the nucleus pulposus. This can result in low back pain.

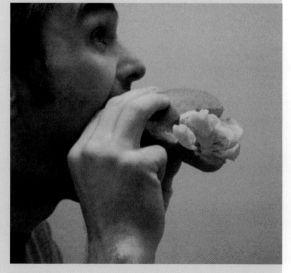

Figure 6.14 • Stress of eating a burger: practical activity 6.2.

draw back their catapult ready to launch another attack. We call this elastic energy and we will return to it in Chapter 9 as it is well used by the body to help propel itself forwards when moving.

Compressive strain occurs due to compressive stress. The stress acts on the body to reduce its size. Calculating this is a little trickier than tensile. Imagine you find a bit of children's play putty and you try to get it back in its container, except it is already full so you first need to make some space in the container by pushing down (compressing) (see Fig. 6.15).

Let's say the height of the putty in the container before was 10 cm. You press down and it reduces to 8 cm. There was a 2-cm reduction in height. Compressive strain is therefore 2 cm/10 cm giving 20% but this is a negative value, since it reduced in size. Try Practical Activity 6.3 to understand the energy in compression.

Like shear stress, shear strain is more difficult to describe. It is measured by the amount of slide that occurs between the layers. This would be an extraordinarily difficult thing to measure at each layer so the body is regarded as one. The strain is more or less regarded as the overall change in angle of the body due to the displacement (slide) of all the layers (see Fig. 6.18).

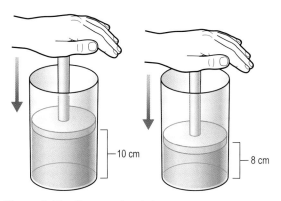

Figure 6.15 • Compressive strain.

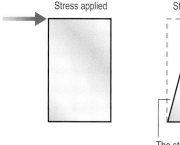
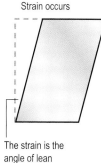

Figure 6.18 • Shear strain.

Practical Activity Box 6.3

Energy from compression

There is also energy stored due to compression. Get a bicycle pump (a syringe would also work). Put your finger over the end of the pump and press the piston in. What you are doing is compressing the air; the movement of the chamber is the compressive strain. When you can go no further take your hand off the piston.

energy within the compressed air. The same effect works for a bouncing ball. As it collides with the ground, the force compresses the ball. This energy is then released to push it into the air. Similar mechanisms are used in some human movement; see Chapter 9.

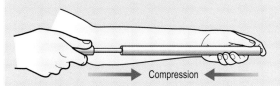

Figure 6.16 • Compressing a bicycle pump.

What you should have found was that the piston bounced back. This is due to the stored potential

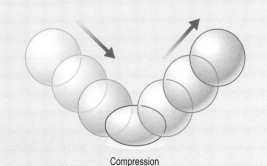

Figure 6.17 • Compression of a bouncing ball.

So, we now understand stress, which is kind of like force, and strain, which is the change in shape of the body, compressed, lengthened or distorted in some way. The way that a material strains when stressed will depend on the many things: how much material there is, what the material consists of at a microscopic level and how that is organized. Clearly it is important to understand this relationship between stress and strain. It can tell us why and how the material will break down and how we can best restore its function.

Stress–strain relationship and stiffness

OK, let's get that elastic band back (unless you broke it with too much stress). We are going to be a bit more empirical (measure things) here and plot a graph. You probably don't have any instruments to measure the amount of stress we will apply but you can measure strain with a ruler. Put your finger through one end of the elastic band onto the ruler so that this end of the rubber band is fixed. Hold the other end with your other hand. Record the length when you are just holding it, pulling slightly perhaps to straighten out any folds. We are now going to explore the stress–strain relationship by pulling the elastic band (see Fig. 6.19).

But first, in the absence of proper instruments we have to come up with a way of quantifying (putting a number to it) how much pull (tensile stress) we apply. How about using food analogies? So apply the following stresses to the elastic and record the length of the elastic band at each stress application in a table that looks like Table 6.1.

Table 6.1 Recording the stress strain relationship

Stress	Strain (increase in length)
1	1 cm
2	
3	
4	

Stress 1: Pull on the elastic band with the amount you would need to pull apart a soft peeled banana.

Stress 2: Pull on the elastic band with the amount you would need to pull apart a piece of cooked pasta.

Stress 3: Pull on the elastic band with the amount you would need to pull apart a French baguette.

Stress 4: Pull on the elastic band with the amount you would need to pull apart the skin of a baked potato.

If you then plot these values you might get something that looks like Figure 6.20. In Figure 6.20 stress has been plotted up the Y axis and strain along the X axis. Remember that strain has been converted into a percentage, the change in length divided by the original length and multiplied by 100. If you join up the points you will have constructed a stress–strain curve. These curves are the cornerstone of material science and the subject of a lot of research. They provide lots of information about a material. First they tell you the **stiffness** of a material. **Stiffness** is a word used generally to mean inflexibility. It's more or less used in the same

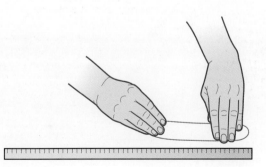

Figure 6.19 ● Stress–strain relationship with an elastic band.

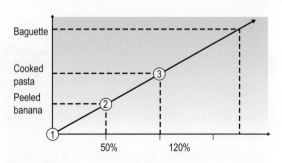

Figure 6.20 ● Hypothetical stress–strain graph of elastic band.

way in material science but has a more precise definition. It is the ratio between stress and strain, i.e.:

$$\textbf{Striffness} = \frac{\textbf{Stress}}{\textbf{Strain}}$$

This is also known as the Young modulus and is often represented by the letter E.

For those among you who prefer pictures to equations this ratio is the same as the gradient (angle) of the slope. In Figure 6.21 there are three stress–strain curves including our rubber band. The higher the slope, the stiffer the material because there is less movement along the X axis (strain) for the same or greater stress (movement up the Y axis). So material A is stiffer than B and B is stiffer than C (which could be our rubber band).

Of course it's impossible to calculate this ratio when your stress is the amount to break cooked spaghetti! The CD-ROM contains an interactive activity that explores stress strain further—see CD-ROM activity 6.1.

Let's look again at a typical stress strain. The graph in Figure 6.22 is the stress–strain graph of a copper

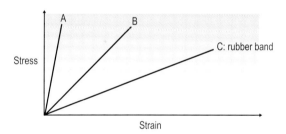

Figure 6.21 • Stress–strain plots of materials with different stiffness values.

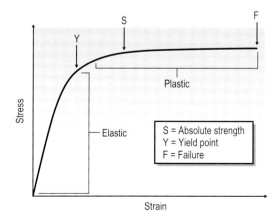

Figure 6.22 • Stress–strain curve of a copper wire.

wire. As you can see the graph has two different slopes divided around the point Y. This is the yield point when the material starts to give; it is essentially tearing. Before this point the material is undamaged and if you stopped stressing it before the yield point it will return to its original shape and properties: this is the **elastic** phase. The change in length during this period is down to separation at atomic level. The bonds weaken a little or may separate, allowing some movement, but not a great deal. So the slope is higher at this stage, more stiff.

After the yield point the material behaves differently; this is the **plastic** phase. The material behaves a little like **plasticene** in this phase: it has lost a lot of its stiffness, allowing quite a lot of lengthening and, like plasticene, it won't return to its original shape or properties when you remove the stress. If you stress material beyond the yield point into the plastic phase you have basically damaged it, broken atomic bonds beyond repair; it won't be the same again.

The way that stress is applied will influence the stress–strain relationship. In particular how fast it is applied alters the stiffness of the material. To understand the effect of time let's conduct a short experiment.

Get a cheap plastic shopping bag and hold it in both hands. Now pull as quickly as you can, i.e. apply a rapid tensile stress. If you are strong enough and the bag cheap enough you should be able to tear the bag. Now get another bag and perform the same movement only this time do it slowly, building up the strength of your pull. This time you should find that the bag lengthens (or strains) more.

So, why did the bag strain more when the stress was applied slowly? The answer lies in something called **viscosity**. This relates to the ability of all materials to **flow**: the **more** viscous, the **less** its ability to flow. Water is not very viscous, steel is highly viscous (but it can still flow!). Without getting too involved in the chemistry it's to do with how strongly the molecules in the material are bonded together as well as how closely packed together they are.

When materials (gases and fluids included) flow they do so by one layer gliding over the other; see

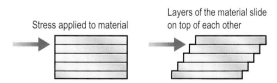

Figure 6.23 • Layers of a material glide (flow) on each other.

Figure 6.23. This is called laminar flow (think of a steady stream from a tap) as opposed to turbulent flow where the layers all mix up (like a tap turned on full or the white water of a river). We are going to talk a lot more about fluids later in Chapter 8.

The ability to flow is an important feature of materials and one you can exploit when trying to stretch out bubble gum or a muscle (we will start talking about human tissues soon as all this food talk can be distracting). The plastic bag demonstrated its viscosity when you applied the stress slowly: the material literally flowed. Of course you wouldn't want too much flowing in your plastic bag; otherwise, you would be dragging your shopping bags along the ground by the time you got home. Of course it would be advisable to use paper bags which are more viscous (i.e. won't flow) and more environmentally friendly!

A few other properties of materials

Another important characteristic of materials and one critical to engineering is **fatigue**. You may have heard of metal fatigue in relation to a building or the wings of an aircraft which are constantly checked for signs of fatigue. Fatigue is structural damage (which can be minor, e.g. microscopic splits) resulting from repetitive application of stress. This is analogous to stress fractures in a sportsman.

   Material strength: this is the amount of stress a material can endure before breaking. It is also known as the absolute strength (see Fig. 6.22) and is essentially the highest point in a stress–strain graph.

   Thixotropy: this is a really interesting property of materials and one that many sports and rehabilitation practitioners can exploit (even unwittingly), so pay attention.

I am sure you have all struggled to get that last bit of tomato sauce stuck at the bottom of the bottle. You try to use gravity by tipping it up but nothing is moving, so you give it a good shake and tip it up again. This time it begins to flow. The sauce has become **less resistant** to flow (i.e. less viscous) out the bottle, because you agitated it. This property of the sauce is called thixotropy and is not just a special property of sticky sauces. In fact, most materials behave in this way *to some degree*. What is happening is that the energy you have transferred

to the material by shaking has unbonded molecules and possibly uncurled coils of long chain molecules, making them more able to slide against one another, so the layers move on top of each other more easily. Put another way there is less friction between the layers. There are lots of materials that behave in this manner. Clay for example is thixotropic which poses problems for houses made of clay especially during an earthquake. The walls of a shaking house will soon start to slide down.

The word thixotropy comes from the Greek words 'thixis', which means to touch/manipulate, and 'tropy', which means to change. So thixotropic means a substance that changes due to being handled.

Of course another way to make a material flow more easily is to heat it up. This is still thixotropy. If you get a bit of sticky tack in your hand and start to roll it around in your hand it will soon become more malleable. This property may not always be desirable. The steel cables in a bridge would be useless if they started to strain more easily in summer. Tarmac that starts to flow in the warm weather can play havoc with traffic. So you have to know if the material you are interested in changes viscosity when heated. But there are obvious advantages: just think of the difference in your flexibility after a warm bath compared to when you wake up after a night camping in the Scottish Highlands, we will talk more about the advantages in the next chapter.

What you need to remember from all that

Materials are not rigid; they change shape (strain) when force (or rather stress) is applied. Stress can be applied in different directions: compressive which squashes, tensile which stretches, shear which crumples and torsional which twists the material. These stresses can exist at the same time; e.g. if a beam bends you get a combination of compressive, tensile and shear stresses. Strain is the amount that the material changes shape as a result of the stress.

The amount of stress needed to cause a certain amount of strain tells you how **stiff** a material is. Stiffness is the ratio between stress and strain, or stress divided by strain. This is also known as the modulus of elasticity or Young's modulus.

If a material returns to the same shape after a stress was applied then the stress was within the material's elastic phase; if more stress is applied and the material changes shape on release then the stress was in the plastic range. So there is a limit to applying stress, after which the material will undergo permanent change. This limit is also called the yield point.

When stress is applied to materials over time then the material is allowed to flow. This depends on its viscosity (resistance to flow), which can change with temperature and agitation (thixotropy). Some materials flow more easily than others.

We have talked about materials in general but what are the materials that make up our bodies? What they are made from and how they behave when loaded is exactly what we are going to cover in the next chapter.

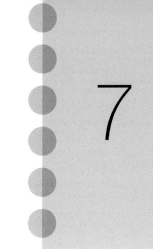

Chapter Seven

Composition and Mechanical Properties of Connective Tissue

What you will learn about in this chapter

1. What connective tissue is and what it is made from;
2. How connective tissue responds to force applications;
3. Structure and mechanical properties of skin, tendon, bone and articular cartilage;
4. How the properties of tissue change with ageing, immobility and injury; and
5. A greater insight into the science of stretching tissues.

Words you will come across

Connective tissue, collagen, ground substance, fibroblasts, ageing, creep, stress, relaxation, immobility, stretching.

In the last chapter we covered a lot of new principles and new words about material science. These were borrowed from the world of engineering (via the Greek language) but let's not forget what we came here for and why you are studying biomechanics. The human body is built from a range of different tissues, some highly specialized like the brain and eye, others more basic (if you can call them that) like ligament and skin. The ways these materials behave is not so dissimilar to what we talked about in the last chapter, with some obvious differences, such as the ability to repair itself. So let's get on with talking about the materials that make up the human body, in particular the ones that provide the mechanical structure for posture and movement.

The structure and strength of the body comes from connective tissue. This includes a range of materials such as bone, tendon, ligament, capsule and skin. Connective tissue also provides the strength and structure for our organs such as the pericardium of the heart or the walls of blood vessels and lungs. In this chapter, however, we will focus on the dense connective tissues of the musculoskeletal system, what it consists of and how it behaves when stressed.

Connective tissue

Connective tissue contains three basic ingredients that vary in amount according to the function of the structure.

Ground substance

This is a shapeless gelatinous goo that surrounds the connective tissue fibres and cells. It is a loose combination of carbohydrates, proteins and water (lots of water). The purpose of this goo is both to nourish and to lubricate the connective tissue, so that the fibres can easily slide over each other. It is the ground substance that gives the connective tissues its viscous (and thixotropic) properties.

Fibres

There are two main fibres in connective tissue: collagen and elastin, with collagen the most prevalent.

Collagen fibres

The word derives from the Greek word for glue (Kolla) and source (gen). So, literally it is the substance that gives us glue (after it has been boiled up!). As well as producing glue, boiling up collagen also gives us gelatin, the basic ingredient of those delicious gummy sweeties. It's the conversion of collagen to gelatin when you roast some meat that makes the meat tender. Collagen is also now widely used for a variety of beauty treatments, e.g. plumping up lips and smoothing wrinkles. Useful stuff indeed.

There are many types of collagen (approximately 28) although most are classified into four types (see Table 7.1 for details). They are constructed slightly differently from each other according to the type of function they perform. The basic unit of collagen is the tropocollagen molecule; this is formed from three intertwined polypeptide chains (Figure 7.1) which are a series of joined-up proteins. The best way to describe how the collagen fibres are constructed from this basic unit is to liken it to how rope is constructed. The basic units of rope (either threads of cotton, hemp or jute) are bunched together into yarns. The yarns (usually there are three, although bigger ropes may use more yarns) are then twisted together to make the rope (see Fig. 7.2). So the strength of rope comes from the way it is woven together; individual threads may break but the rope will still be intact.

Collagen is more or less the same: tropocollagen fibres bunched into microfibrils, which are organized

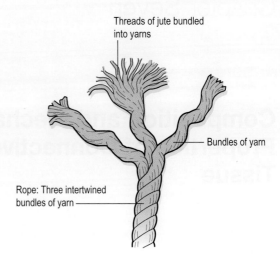

Figure 7.2 • Rope is made from intertwined bundles of thread.

into subfibrils and ultimately the rope of collagen is finished. A notable difference between rope and collagen is that at the subfibril level of organization the gooey substance (ground substance) separates the subfibrils. This confers mechanical qualities on collagen different than those of rope, giving it a greater ability to flow when placed under stress. We will talk more about this later.

The organized structure of collagen gives connective tissue its shape and a lot of its strength. Of course it varies in amount according to how strong the tissue has to be. So tissue requiring a lot of strength, such as tendon, will have a lot of collagen tightly packed together, whereas other tissues that do not have to accommodate these large stresses will have less collagen and perhaps be more loosely organized.

Elastic fibres

Connective tissue also must be elastic; to stretch a little when stressed and be able to return to normal when the stress is removed. Although collagen has some elastic qualities a lot of the elastic properties of connective tissue come from the elastic fibres. These fibres are present in many connective tissues in varying amounts depending on how much elasticity is required. Think about all the bits of your body that are repeatedly stretched and then immediately return to their original size, e.g. skin, lungs and blood vessels.

Can you think of any other part of the body that regularly undergoes a change in shape before snapping back?

Elastic fibres are primarily made of bundles of elastin, which is a kind of coil of various amino

Table 7.1 Main types of collagen		
Type	**Location**	**Function**
1	Tendon, skin, artery walls, scar tissue, bones	Tensile strength and shape
2	Articular cartilage, fibrocartilage	Strength, including shear and compression
3	Granulation tissue	Early scaffold during tissue repair
4	Lens of eye and basal membrane	Structure and strength

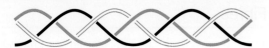

Figure 7.1 • Intertwining tropocollagen molecule.

acids. This coiled shape mean the fibres will return to their original shape after being stretched. You could think of them as small, but fairly weak springs. They can be arranged either in a haphazard manner or more regularly according to the direction that they are regularly stretched in, which will depend on the function of the tissue. For example skin requires elasticity in many different directions, whereas a tendon has a more consistent direction of stretch along the direction of the muscle pull.

The cells

Finally there are three main cells in connective tissue which perform a range of functions critical to the health and continued development of the tissue. These cells are:

1. Fibroblasts, which produce the fibres and ground substance;

2. Macrophages, which are phagocytes, basically little cannibals going around eating up any dead cells and other debris resulting from infection or tissue damage; and

3. Neutrophils (white blood cells), which are the cells which arrive first at a site of infection attacking and neutralizing microbes; some types of white blood cells produce the necessary antibodies to fight infection.

So, these basic constituents of connective tissue appear in different amounts and arrangements in our connective tissues, in the same way that different amounts and types of wood might be used in the construction of a building. Like collagen in the human body, the core material is the same throughout. The steel used to make the spring in a child's toy has been worked into a specific shape but it is still the same steel used in the construction of an aeroplane. The same material in different volumes and shape serves many different functions.

With this in mind let's look at some of the main bits of connective tissue in a bit more detail starting with the largest part of our musculoskeletal system, the skin.

Skin

It might be worth starting this section with a quick demonstration. Straighten your arm out with palm up. Now pinch about 1 cm of the skin on your forearm and pull it so that your skin lifts a little from your arm, but not enough that it hurts you. Now let go. You applied a tensile force to the skin and on release it immediately returned to its shape without any harm. This is elasticity. Try to do the same thing at different locations on your forearm and try different directions of pull. Neither should matter: your skin will always snap back when you remove the stress no matter which direction you pulled in. This means the mechanical property of skin is isotropic: it's the same regardless of direction. Anisotropic is where the strength and elasticity is better one direction than another.

Understanding the ability of the skin to recoil after being stretched has obvious implications for professionals working in burns and plastics as well as cosmetic surgery. However, it is also relevant to those of you interested in increasing joint flexibility. Afterall the skin around a joint must be flexible enough for the joint to move.

To demonstrate this grab a handful (well as much you can) of the skin on the front of your elbow while it is bent. Now try to straighten it. Inextensible scar tissue will behave in a similar way to restrict joint movement. You may also be interested in understanding how skin can be injured during sports participation. The skin on the sole of the feet, for example, experiences large compressive and shear forces during many sports. Of course the same could be said for the hands during racket sports, rowing, rock climbing etc. There are lots of relevance, so let's get on with what skin is made of and what its function is.

Skin has three layers: the epidermis, dermis and hyodermis. The topmost layer, the epidermis, is mainly concerned with providing a protective (and weatherproof) barrier for the body, rather like a biological Gore-Tex.

Beneath the epidermis lies the dermis; this is where the real mechanical characteristics of skin are contained. As well as glands and hair follicles the dermis contains an irregular pattern of dense connective tissue. Its irregularity is important as skin needs strength and elasticity in different directions—isotropy. So no matter which way it is pulled and pushed it will have the same strength. The final layer, the hyodermis, is a transient layer that connects the skin to the underlying fat tissue.

The fat underneath skin is not just to keep you warm in winter; it also has some mechanical properties, particularly in coping with compressive stress on the tissue. This is best illustrated by the

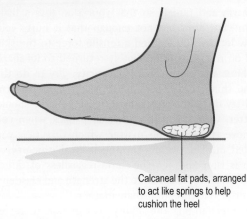

Calcaneal fat pads, arranged to act like springs to help cushion the heel

Figure 7.3 ● Calcaneal fat pads at heel strike.

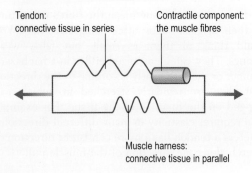

Tendon: connective tissue in series

Contractile component: the muscle fibres

Muscle harness: connective tissue in parallel

Figure 7.4 ● Hill's model of muscle.

calcaneal fat pads, which are positioned under the heel to perform like springs when the heel strikes the ground during the gait cycle (see Fig. 7.3), allowing some cushioning to parts of the body which experience large compressive stresses, a bit like the springs in a mattress.

Muscle

Experiments have demonstrated that the structure most likely to cause a loss of flexibility at a joint is the muscle; shortened muscles are a frequent companion to many clinical conditions such as arthritis and stroke as well as affecting performance in sport and creating risk of further injury. Therefore, it is worth spending a little time on the structure of muscle, and in particular the connective tissue components.

Muscle can be separated into two different functional parts. The contractile part and the connective tissue part, which gives the muscle its passive mechanical properties. The contractile component is the part that creates tension within the muscle through the bonding and unbonding of the myosin protein onto the actin protein. This tension is translated to the bone via the tendon.

The connective tissue in muscle is in two places. At the end of the muscle there is connective tissue, i.e. the tendon, which is also called series connective tissue because it is at the end. The other part of the muscle made of connective tissue is the muscle harness. This is made of sheaths of connective that wrap around the contractile component; this is sometimes called the parallel connective tissue. This structure of muscle is shown diagrammatically

in Figure 7.4. Because it was first described by the English physiologist Archibald Vivian Hill in 1938 it is known as Hill's model of muscle.

Connective tissue in series: the tendon

The primary function of a tendon is to transfer the pulling force of a muscle to the attached bone. This may be to create a turning force large enough to move a joint through an arc of movement or enough tension to maintain a bone's position whilst another part of the body performs an action.

In accordance with the principle that the shape and structure of a tissue is dictated by its function (form follows function), the collagen fibres of muscle tendon are both densely packed in (to provide strength) and arranged in straight lines according to the direction of the tensile stresses placed on the tendon (see Figure 7.5) from the pull of muscle.

You may have noticed in Figure 7.5 that although the collagen fibres are lined up parallel to each other, they are wavy and not straight at all. This wavy pattern has been widely reported in connective and is called the 'crimp'. It creates a specific feature of the stress–strain relationship which we will talk about shortly. A tendon is not only required to be strong enough to cope with the tensile forces from muscle contractions, it also needs to allow some strain and be able to recover or recoil, i.e. elasticity. This is an important characteristic as it allows

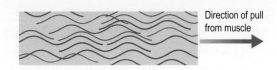

Direction of pull from muscle

Figure 7.5 ● Collagen arrangement in tendon.

the muscle–tendon unit to absorb some of the forces applied to the body (otherwise, it would be in danger of snapping) and then reuse this stored energy as the tendon (and muscle harness) return to their original shape.

Elastic energy storage and release has become an important observation of the way the musculoskeletal system functions. Although difficult to measure in living humans this property has been estimated to contribute up to 60% of the mechanical work of walking with the elastic energy stored primarily in the Achilles tendon (Chapter 9 develops this idea further).

This ability of tendons to strain (lengthen) means that when you apply a passive stretch to a muscle around 50% of any change in overall muscle length (of course this will vary across tendons) will occur at the tendon; something to think about when you are next stretching someone's muscle.

The only way to answer the questions in Practical Activity Box 7.1 is to look at the stress–strain relationship of human tendon through experiments like our stress–strain experiment on p. 84. Experiments on human tissue are typically done on dead tissue

(for obvious reasons); nevertheless they offer rich information that can be very useful for those of you engaged in improving flexibility as well as restoring muscle function.

Figure 7.7 shows a typical stress–strain relationship for human tendon; it does resemble the

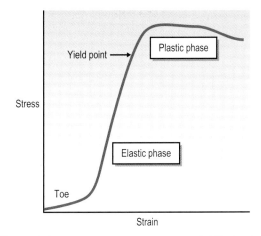

Figure 7.7 • Stress–strain graph of a human Achilles tendon.

Practical Activity Box 7.1

As we have said, being at the end of the muscle the tendon will experience large amounts of tensile stress. Take the gluteus medius (hip abductor) tendon for example (see Figure 7.6). Stand up and abduct your leg (lift your leg out to the side). The muscle shortens, thanks to the contractile component; this pulls on the tendon which is fixed to the greater trochanter of the femur. This force overcomes the leg's inertia and it lifts up. As the leg lifts off the ground, the muscle then must create forces to contend with the adducting moment caused by the mass of the leg (centred approximately at the knee) moving out to the side away from the hip joint.

Now keep your leg out to the side, just like the plastic bags containing your shopping (see p. 86). You don't want your tendon to start lengthening despite the tensile stress from the muscle pulling it up and the leg pulling it down. The tendon must be stiff enough to resist this persistent tensile stress. How much more stress can the tendon take? Would it make any difference if you performed the movement 20 times? And what would happen if you held it there for 15 minutes (aside from the muscle fatigue)?

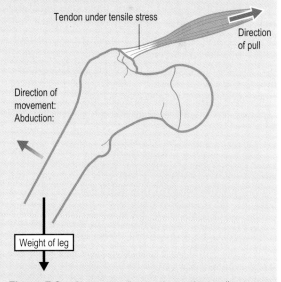

Figure 7.6 • Gluteus medius tendon under tensile stress.

stress–strain relationships of other materials, e.g. copper wire (p. 85, Fig. 6.22). It's got a yield point and elastic and plastic phases but it's got extra bits and is more complex. Let's look at it in more detail, starting at the bottom of the slope which is called the toe region.

The toe region is a consistent finding in studies of tendon and ligament in particular but not really found in non-biological tissues. During the toe region there is a less stiff response to stress; i.e. the tissue elongates more easily. It appears that during this phase the tissue loses its crimp (remember that? see Fig. 7.5). It is a bit like pulling the ends of a sheet to stretch it over a bed; in doing this any creases or folds in the sheet smooth out, just like the crimp in connective tissue. Some studies suggest that the force required to uncrimp a tendon is similar to the amount experienced during normal activities. So you can imagine the tissue moving in and out of its wavy pattern as you move around.

The elastic phase is similar to that described for other materials; i.e. as more stress is applied gradually more and more fibres become involved. You could imagine a tug-of-war team. The competitors take up the slack (uncrimping of the toe region), and then as the two teams begin to pull, more and more team members become engaged in the battle; this is the elastic phase. It is important to remember that during these first two phases (toe and elastic) the tissue has not been damaged and that when the stress is taken off the tissue will return to its previous shape AND previous properties; i.e. you haven't changed its shape or weakened it. You can use the slope of the stress–strain curve during the elastic phase to calculate the stiffness of the tendon, dividing stress by strain.

The curve begins to change at the yield point. We have reached the point where damage to fibres is taking place and the tissue begins to lose its ability to resist the stress. Like in an Indiana Jones film with the hero halfway across the bridge and the rope begins to fray and unwind, he knows there is only a little time left before the bridge breaks and he plummets to the ground. The tendon is no different: continue to apply the stress and the tendon will break. After the yield point, if you take the stress away the tissue will be permanently damaged (well at least until it repairs itself). It is weaker, less stiff and possibly longer. Of course making the tissue longer may be your intention, which we'll talk a bit more about at the end of this chapter and again in Chapter 10.

Connective tissue in parallel: the muscle harness

Muscle harness may not be an expression you are familiar with but it is a useful way of describing the connective tissue which surrounds the contractile units in parallel, as opposed to tendon, which is at the end of muscle (i.e. in series). In yet another well-organized structure muscle fibres are parceled together by connective tissue into fascicles; groups of fascicles are then held together by more connective tissue (the endomysium), which are further bunched into larger groups by yet more connective tissue (the perimysium). Finally a sheath of connective tissue surrounds the whole muscle; this is the epimysium. Together all this connective tissue makes up the muscle harness. The word harness is useful here because it holds the muscle together and helps channel the force created by the muscle—just like a horse's harness. In many ways it behaves like the tendon; although strength is its main attribute, the muscle harness also behaves viscoelastically, i.e. it can flow when stressed over time and returns to its original shape when stress is removed.

Bone

Let's move on to bone. This is a really interesting biological material, providing rigidity to our body, protection to our vital organs, body and rigid beams for our muscles to create and control movement. These are just their mechanical functions. Within bone there is storage space for calcium, red and white blood cells and platelets, all vital to the health and function of our body. However, as this is a book about biomechanics let's concentrate on the mechanical properties of bone.

There are all sorts of types of bones in your body, and lots of them (> 200). We can't look at them all so we will consider a typical long bone like the femur and uncover some of its makeup so that we can understand its mechanical properties. But first let's start with the basic composition of bone.

Bone is primarily formed from osseous (another word for bone) tissue, which is made from a combination of collagen and hard minerals (calcium, magnesium and phosphate), which make the bone pretty rigid. Bone tissue is arranged into two broad types.

Spongy or cancellous bone (also called trabecular) is situated on the inside of a bone. It is arranged into a network of struts, a bit like scaffolding (except on the inside). Because of this arrangement it is very light (only around 20% of total bone mass) but crucially it is still strong. This design has been imitated by many engineers. You only need to glance at the Forth Road bridge in Edinburgh to see this. Perhaps there are buildings or bridges in your area that imitate the crisscross struts of cancellous bone.

Hard compact tissue provides the white outer layer of bone, surrounding the cancellous bone. It is very dense so it is a very tough structure, good for withstanding impacts as well as the pull of muscles, so this part of the bone is protective; see Figure 7.8. When you think about it the structure of bone is a bit like a Malteser chocolate sweet: a shell of hard compact chocolate on the outside and a light honeycomb inside, i.e. lots of little struts.

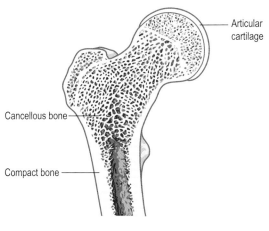

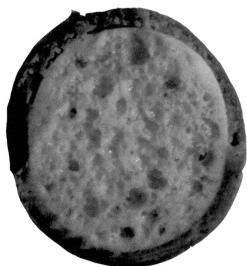

Figure 7.8 • Types of bone and a Malteser.

So, what are the mechanical properties of bone?

The compact layer (hard outer shell) makes bone very tough, great for resisting direct blows (to protect your internal organs), as well as shear and bending stress from external forces and the pull of tendons and ligaments. The matrix network of the cancellous bone means it is light (essential for efficient movement); however, because it is constructed from minerals, as well as collagen, it is rigid, making it very good at resisting compressive forces without deforming (afterall you don't want to shrink when you stand up). Bone is not so good, however, at resisting tensile forces and because of its high mineral content is relatively brittle; i.e. although it has high strength it cannot flow like tendon and skin, so cannot absorb a lot of energy. It is therefore more prone to complete disruption—fracture.

Articular cartilage

At the ends of bone is the articular cartilage. Articular cartilage is a highly specialized connective tissue constructed from chondrocytes (cartilage cells), collagen and water. It doesn't include either blood vessels or nerves. It has three main functions:

- Withstand compressive loading;
- Distribute load; and
- Decrease friction.

It achieves these functions with its structure which echoes that of skin. It is arranged into four zones. The top zone (tangential layer) has loads of water and fine collagen fibres weaved parallel to the surface (and like skin, in different directions). The chondrocytes are flat and packed reasonably close together. The orientation of collagen is important to cope with the shear forces as the bones glide on top of each other. The high water content in this zone helps to reduce friction, in the same way that a layer of water in an ice hockey rink makes it even more slippery.

In the next zone (transition layer), the collagen fibres become less parallel and the chondrocytes more rounded. This helps the tissue to cope more with compressive forces. The third zone (radial layer) is engineered to absorb a lot of the compressive strain, e.g. from weight bearing, with the chondrocytes arranged vertically into columns or stacks and collagen fibres lined up along side them. The final zone (calcified cartilage) marks the transition between cartilage and bone (see Fig. 7.9).

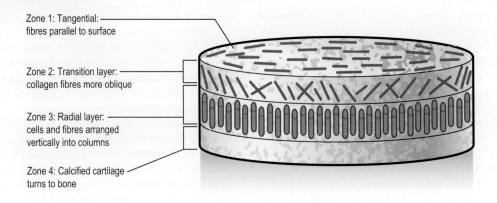

Zone 1: Tangential:
fibres parallel to surface

Zone 2: Transition layer:
collagen fibres more oblique

Zone 3: Radial layer:
cells and fibres arranged
vertically into columns

Zone 4: Calcified cartilage
turns to bone

Figure 7.9 • Zones of articular cartilage.

Tissue remodelling

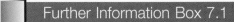

One of the most fascinating aspects of bone (and indeed all connective tissue) is its ability to remodel. This ability was first described in bone and was called Wolff's law after the nineteenth-century Austrian physician Julius Wolff. Basically the law states that bones adapt (throughout life) to the forces placed on them. Bone tissue is constantly being created and re-absorbed; this is called bone turnover. It's a bit like filling a bath with the plug out. As you pour water in it drains away down the plug. A point can be reached where the amount of water going into the bath equals the amount going out and so the water level remains the same. You could change this level by turning the taps or changing the size of the plug. In the same way bone can readily adapt to a change in the forces it habitually experiences by increasing (opening the tap and closing the plug) or decreasing (closing the tap and opening the plug) the amount of bone tissue.

If you place more stress on your right arm, for example through taking up javelin throwing or ten pin bowling, then the bones of the right side will adapt to these additional forces by laying down more bone tissue (as well as muscle). Of course the opposite can also happen. A decrease in force, e.g. having your arm in a sling, will trigger a reduction in bone density (the plug opens more and the tap closes a little) see Further Information Box 7.2 to see how Astronauts coped with this. This ability of bone became evident through careful examination of the cadavers of different people, modern and ancient (see Further Information Box 7.1).

This turnover of bone tissue has more that one purpose, however. It also helps to regulate the level

Further Information Box 7.1

The field of palaeopathology has profited greatly by this ability of bone. This is a field of archaeology that concerns itself with studying human (and animal) skeletal remains, looking for signs of disease (like arthritis) as well as patterns of bone formation that might give clues on the individual's occupation; e.g. degeneration of the lower back might indicate someone involved in a lot of lifting. These skeletal markers of occupational stress have been used to identify people who used a hoe for farming due to the overdevelopment of the bone where the toe flexors attach, indicating that these muscles were very strong, which might have resulted from a lot of spade work. Similar approaches have been used to identify archers and hunters.

of calcium in the body: too much and it stores it, too little and it releases some from its store. Bone turnover is also important in the repair of damaged bone tissue. Bone is laid down at the site of damage (like a fracture) until the structure becomes stable again before proceeding onto a process of reduction and remodelling.

The same thing occurs in other connective tissue, skin, tendon, etc. These tissues are smart; they sense that more strength is required to cope with a change in the force experienced and make the appropriate increase in amount and organization of the collagen fibres.

This ability of connective tissue to adapt to the forces they routinely experience is constantly exploited by sports and rehabilitation professionals. We will talk about this in more detail in Chapter 10 but for now think about what you are doing to connective tissue when you alter someone's posture, increase the volume of an athlete's training or place insoles in a shoe to alter the pattern of pressure in their feet.

There are a number of factors which affect the properties of connective tissue. In this next bit we are going to look at the effects of immobility, maturation, ageing, stretching and temperature.

Inactivity (immobilization)

We have already mentioned the role that activity/exercise has on connective tissue. The forces produced by activity provide the stimulus for bone growth, but what happens if you, or part of you such as your arm or leg, are prevented from being active?

When immobilized, muscle quickly adapts to the position it is kept in. It does this by altering the number of muscle fibres (the contractile part) it has in series, the number of links in the chain, like the captain of a tug-of-war team putting more or less men (or women) into the team, so it is longer or shorter. Basically, if a muscle is immobilized in its shortened position it will decrease in length. The other connective tissues also adapt. Without the guiding stimulus of force, any new collagen produced in ligaments and tendons will be arranged haphazardly, less dense

and less regular. Think of a squadron of soldiers on parade. While on parade they are all lined up, strong and organized. On the signal to dismiss they fall apart, move off in different directions. Similarly connective tissue becomes weak, and also less flexible. This may seem a contradiction (weak and stiff) but the stiffness develops from more cross connections between the fibres as well as a loss of water in the ground substance through lack of movement. Experiments have demonstrated that this weak and stiff connective tissue resulting from immobilization takes up to 18 months to be fully restored.

Factors that make immobilization worse are:

1. Prolonged and complete immobilization;

2. Immobilization following an injury, particularly if there is still swelling; and

3. If the immobilized person is old.

Maturation

As children mature, the stability of the bonds within the tropocollagen molecules in collagen increases. Stronger bonds make the collagen more resistant to tensile stress. There are also increasing amounts of cross-linking between collagen fibres as the child grows, which further strengthens the connective tissue but makes it less flexible. Musculoskeletal tissue in children is typically more compliant because of the greater water of the ground substance as well as having immature collagen fibres. I am sure we can all identify with a decrease in flexibility since childhood.

Effect of ageing

The effect of ageing on connective tissue is actually quite similar to the effects of disuse; indeed some people have argued that it is not ageing in itself but rather reduced levels of activity in older people that cause more deterioration.

Generally speaking as we age there is a decrease in collagen turnover (creation and absorption of collagen). Collagen becomes thinner and is present in reduced amounts. The collagen fibres also become more attached to each other—cross links, which can be helpful in stiffening up materials but also prevent them straining. This is compounded by a loss of water content in ground substance which makes the tissue less capable of elongating.

Practical Activity Box 7.2

Ageing as a dried banana skin

Next time you eat a banana keep the skin and put it on a cloth to dry. At first the skin is compliant: you can stretch it nicely; it will break but can take quite a bit of stress first. Leave it for a week or so (don't worry about the smell; it will add a wholesome organic aroma). Now try to stretch it, it won't give (stiff) and will break easily. I am not saying this is exactly what happens to tissue from ageing and immobilization but it has similarities.

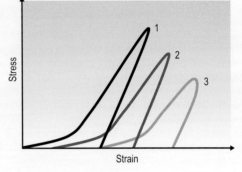

Figure 7.10 • Cyclical loading of connective tissue.

Further Information Box 7.3

Ehlers Danlos disease is caused by an alteration in the process of constructing collagen fibres. There is less collagen produced and it is of poorer quality. Consequently connective tissue is weak and easily deformed. This means joints are hyper-flexible (hypermobile) and the skin is extremely stretchy. This can result in premature degeneration of the musculoskeletal system (e.g. osteoarthritis) and predispose the individual to joint dislocations and other injuries. In its most severe presentation Ehlers Danlos can cause premature death due to the damage of major blood vessels weakened by the lack of strength from good-quality collagen.

Consequently tissue becomes weaker and less able to lengthen. That is, it is more brittle, less able to absorb energy (try Practical Activity 7.2). However, just like immobilized tissue these changes can be reversed, to some degree. For example one study in 2003 demonstrated a 65% improvement in stiffness following 14 weeks of exercise.

Effect of recent history (for example, stretching before a game)

It is traditional and globally observed that athletes stretch before a sporting activity, particularly if the activity requires agility like gymnastics. Reasons given for doing this include:

1. Improved performance;
2. Prevention of injury during the game; and
3. Prevention of longer-term injury.

Although this seems intuitive there is very little evidence supporting these claims; indeed there is evidence to contradict them. However, stretching before participation in sport does seem sensible; perhaps it was ingrained into us at an early age. So let's take a scientific look at this problem by looking at the effect stretching has on the stress–strain relationship. Although taken mainly from animal studies it appears that repetition, or cyclical loading of tissue causes a gradual decrease in stiffness and strength. It becomes more compliant, but weaker.

Figure 7.10 demonstrates this effect. Stretches 2 and 3 show greater amount of strain (moves further along the Y axis) but are able to contend with less stress (lower on Y axis).

Temperature

Research tells us quite clearly that the **temperature** of the tissue being stressed is important. You probably already knew this from your physical education classes when you went through the routine of warming up before a sport.

When connective tissue is cold there is an increase in the tissue stiffness, probably due to an increase in the viscosity (stiffer) of the ground substance. This is a bit like when you freeze your home-baked bread. Fresh out the oven it is soft and malleable; after a few days in the freezer, however, it is hard and brittle (i.e. it will break without bending) (try Practical Activity 7.3). This happens with cold connective tissue as well: there is an increase in the risk of rupture because the tissue can't give. This quality of connective tissue to alter its viscosity with temperature is called thixotropy, which was introduced in the last chapter (see p. 86).

Practical Activity Box 7.3

Get a lump of sticky tack, like Blu Tack, and cool it down (put it in the freezer for an hour or so). Take it out and try to pull it; you should find that it has become more resistant to stress (stiffer) and will snap apart quite easily. Keep pulling it and playing with it until it warms. After a while you will notice that it will stretch out more easily; i.e. it has become less stiff. Connective tissue has the same property.

On the other hand if you increase the temperature of connective tissue too much the bonds in the tropocollagen helix uncouple. So if you apply stress there will be greater strain and the tissue will reach rupture faster.

Clearly if you increase the temperature of connective tissue too much you will destroy the cells; the damaged tissue will then undergo a process of inflammation and synthesis of new collagen. To do this you need to exceed temperatures of 40°C so don't worry: an exercise-based warm-up will not do this. You would have to do some serious boiling.

You may have noticed that connective tissue responds the same way to an increase in temperature as it does to repetitive loading. This is not a coincidence; exactly the same thing is happening to the tissue due to the energy transfer from the heat or from repetitive movement: a change in viscosity of the ground substance (thixotropy) and possibly a change in the bonds of the tropocollagen molecule. So a moderate increase in connective tissue temperature either from repetitive movement or direct heat source such as a bath will make stretching easier. Let's have a closer look at how we stretch, because we all do it differently.

Science of stretch

It might be a good idea to start this section with a practical exercise, one that demonstrates the difference between creep and stress relaxation. If you really can't be bothered there is a demonstration on your CD-ROM, activity 7.1.

Stand up and place your hands on the front of your thighs. Now keep your knees straight and slide your hands down your legs as far as you can. You will eventually feel a tight uncomfortable feeling in the back of your thighs, which of course indicates that your hamstrings muscles have reached their

maximum length (in a conscious state anyway). Stop at this point and make a mental note of the sensation. This is the physiological length of the muscle. Now hold your hands in the same position and count slowly to 20. By the end of this time you should have felt a marked decrease in the uncomfortable tight feeling. What has happened is there has been a decrease in tension within the muscle. This is called **stress relaxation**.

Now wait 20 minutes or so (in this time you could have a think about why this happened). Why was there a reduction in tension when the muscle was held at its physiological length?

Now repeat the same thing only this time when you feel the tissue decrease in tension stretch down a little further; repeat a couple of times. You should find you are able to reach further down because of an increase in the length of your tissues. This is called **tissue creep**.

In both stress relaxation and creep the same process has occurred: when you reached your limit the collagen fibres were allowed to slide past each other a certain amount. Without further stress this results in a decrease in tension within the muscle (there is also a nerve reflex that helps to relax a tense muscle) so you get that stress relaxation. However, when you decided to keep the stress up, this movement of the collagen fibres manifested in an increase in tissue length; this was the tissue creep. The differences between stress relaxation and creep are demonstrated in Figures 7.11 and 7.12, respectively.

Do you think there are any negative implications for tissue creep and what should you do to keep the tissue healthy and intact (see Appendix 7)?

These changes in the length of tissue due to creep are short-lived, because the collagen begins to revert back to its original shape. Elongation in tissue from creep will last anywhere between 30 and 90 minutes, depending on what you are doing

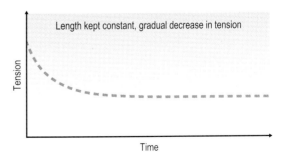

Figure 7.11 • Stress relaxation.

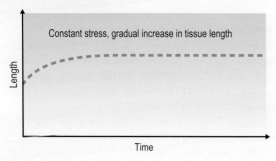

Figure 7.12 • Tissue creep.

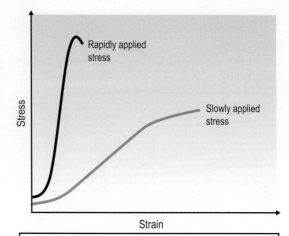

In the rapidly applied stress, although more stress can be applied (higher up the y axis), it reaches the breaking point much sooner. When the stress is applied more slowly the tissue adapts, more strain can be achieved before the yield point is reached.

Figure 7.13 • Response of connective tissue to slow and fast stress application.

during that time. If you are moving around it tends to last longer; complete rest and it will not last as long.

So if you are interested in improving someone's flexibility by increasing the length of the connective tissue, tissue creep is only a short-term solution. To gain a lasting change we need to alter the habitual daily stress the tissue goes through; this means for example the forces a tendon experiences, the range of motion the joint goes through or the length that a muscle is held in, for example while sitting. This is called the tissue's mechanical background and you can alter it by a simple change in someone's sitting posture, tennis serving technique, step length of their gait, etc. Some health and sports professionals impose a change in the tissue's daily stress by using splints or braces that maintain the posture of a joint and therefore the length of surrounding tissue; more on this in Chapter 10.

One thing we haven't talked about is how fast you apply the stretch. Remember the practical activity (p. 85) when you tore the plastic shopping bag. It's the same for connective tissue: if you apply the stress too rapidly it doesn't get a chance to comply to the stress through straining, which absorbs some of the energy. It will therefore reach its yield point rapidly and permanent damage will occur. Applied slowly and the tissue is allowed to give, for the collagen and elastin fibres to take up the strain. A greater increase in length is possible with a slow application of stress before any damage occurs; this is particularly the case with stiffer tissues, e.g. older tissues. See Figure 7.13.

Now, of course, permanently lengthening a tissue may be your aim; in which case a rapidly applied stress, e.g. a physiotherapist or chiropractor manipulating a joint (applying high-velocity thrusting movement to a joint), might be appropriate. However, you need to take account of the fact that damaged tissue will trigger an inflammatory response

with new (potentially stiffer) collagen being laid down. If you do not follow up the manipulation with daily range of movement exercises (changing the mechanical background) to maintain the new length you will quickly be back at the starting point again.

What you need to remember from all that

We have covered a lot of information in this chapter so it is worth recapping on a few important things. Connective tissue consists of ground substance, collagen and elastin fibres and cells that create new fibres and help repair the tissue. The mechanical properties of connective tissue vary according to the amount and organization of collagen which gives the tissue strength, elastin which improves tissue elasticity and the viscosity of ground substance which allows the tissue to flow. These mechanical properties alter with age, physical activity (and immobilization), temperature and recent history.

We know that a warm-up helps tissue elongate by reducing the viscosity of the ground substance; this is achieved through repetitive movement and an increase in temperature. Creep is different from stress relaxation only in that new length is gained with creep while reduced tension is achieved in stress relaxation; otherwise, the mechanism is the same. Increased length from creep lasts only a short period (about the duration of a game of football); to maintain length changes the everyday mechanical background of the tissue must change. Finally we know that connective tissue responds more stiffly to a rapid stress, reaching breaking point quickly, whereas a slowly applied force can gain greater change in length before reaching the point where damage occurs.

Chapter Eight

Flow

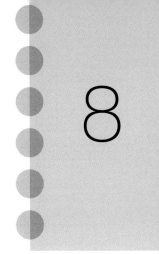

What you will learn about in this chapter

1. Density;
2. Pressure: hydrostatic and atmospheric;
3. How gases and fluids flow;
4. Bernoulli's principle;
5. Drag; and
6. How fluids can be used for exercise.

Words you will come across

Density, relative density, hydrostatic pressure, buoyancy, turbulence, drag.

In the last chapter we talked a bit about how connective tissues flowed. In this chapter (in which you will need at least 5 balloons and 1 bucket) we will take a closer look at flow, but this time thinking more about fluids and gases. Now you might think that this is really the concern of plumbers, nautical engineers and aviators, amongst others, but when you think about it professionals dealing with the human body need to understand how gases and fluids move. After all it is the movement of air around our lungs, blood around our vascular system and spinal fluid around our brain and spinal column that nourishes, protects and sustains our body systems. Outside the body knowledge of flow is critical if you are trying to construct a water-based exercise programme, or you might be working with athletes who participate in speed sports. Understanding air and water flow in this case will help improve performance.

Fluids and gases are forms of matter that continuously change shape when stresses are applied to them. This, theoretically, includes solids like plastic and human connective tissue. In this chapter we will focus on the behaviour of gases and liquids which are surprisingly similar. Afterall, objects can float (or sink) in both liquids and gas and they both create drag, so it is useful to consider them together.

Relative density

Let's begin with floating. To understand why and how some objects float we need to introduce a few principles and definitions, namely **density** and **relative density** (RD). All bodies have **density**, which is the amount of mass confined within its shape or volume of the body. We talked about this in Chapter 2 when we discussed the centre of mass. Density then is simply the mass divided by the volume, i.e.:

$$\text{Density (P)} = \frac{\text{Mass (kg)}}{\text{Volume (m}^3\text{)}}$$

Density tells you how spread out the mass is within the body shape. Liquids have a low density (molecules more spread out) compared to solids; e.g. the density of pure water is 1 g per cubic centimetre (g/cm^3), whereas mercury is more dense (molecules are packed more closely together) with 13.6 g/cm^3. Other notable densities are copper at 8.89 g/cm^3, wood at around 0.5 g/cm^3 (depending on the type) and ice at 0.92 g/cm^3, which,

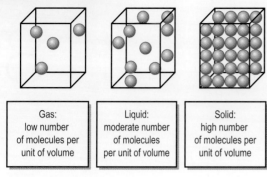

Figure 8.1 ● Density of gases, fluids and solids.

you may note, is lower than pure water. Gases are even less dense. Air for example has a density of 0.0012 g/cm^3. See Figure 8.1 for an illustration of the differences.

Relative density is the ratio between the density of a particular substance and the density of a reference substance. For liquids the reference liquid is pure water (density = 1 g/cm^3) and for gases it is dry air at sea level at a temperature of 20°C (density = 0.0012 g/cm^3). So, for example, the relative density of copper is 8.89; i.e. it is 8.89 times denser than water and 7408 times denser than air.

Anything with a RD > 1 (heavier than pure water) will not float in pure water, so copper will not float, whereas wood (0.5, although this varies with type) will. This value also tells you (as a percentage) how much of the body will be under the water. With a RD of 0.5 a lump of wood will have 50% of its mass under the water. As you may recall ice had a density lower (0.92) than water which is why you only see the tip of the iceberg: 92% under water, 8% above. The human body has a RD a little higher than ice but still less than 1, with a value around 0.96; 4% of the body will float, but which 4%?

🔘 CD-ROM activity 8.1. Floaters and Sinkers

If you try to float in a swimming pool (not exactly pure water but it is difficult and expensive to get enough pure water to float in) you may *not* find that 4% of you floats above the water. You might, instead, sink. The value, 0.96, is an average value and of course people vary. You might even say we can be categorized as sinkers or floaters (try Practical Activity 8.1), depending on whether our densities are above or below that of pure water. The other problem is that this is an overall value for the human body. Different parts of our body have different densities.

Basically your musculoskeletal system, bones, muscles, tendons, etc. are more dense (RD >1); fat is less dense with an RD around 0.9. In addition you retain just over a litre of air in your lungs at all times, which of course means your lungs are much less dense. So if you lie on your back in a swimming pool you will probably find that your legs will sink (lots of bone, tendon and muscle). However, your chest (lots of cavities, fat and air) will float. In fact, because the back of your chest contains the most lung tissue, this is the part which is most likely to float, which is why you see 'dead' people floating on their front in those grisly scenes at the start of crime films. As anyone who has learned to swim will know the mushroom position (face down in water, wrapping your arms around your bent knee) is the most stable position (easiest to maintain) because the 4% that wants to be out of the water (upper back) is out the water; it is not, however, a particularly sustainable position.

Exactly the same principle applies for gases: if you are lighter than the air around you, you will float, heavier and you will sink (or rather you won't float). But don't worry. With a density almost 800 times more than air, there isn't much chance of you spontaneously floating away. Hot moist air is even lighter than normal dry air so it will rise, something the Montgolfier brothers exploited in their early attempt at flight. However, density alone can't explain why planes (which are definitely heavier than air) can stay up in the sky; we also need to understand pressure within fluids and gases and how differences in pressure can cause pulling and lifting forces.

We have already talked a bit about pressure in Chapter 4 when we considered solid bodies in contact with each other, e.g. your feet on the ground. The pressure at your feet was measured as the force divided by the contact area. Pressure within a fluid is not, unfortunately, as easy to measure because there are so many contact points. The stuff just keeps moving about.

Hydrostatic pressure

The molecules in a fluid or gas are not as tightly constrained as they are in solids; they are more free to move around, colliding with each other as they do (Fig. 8.2). These collisions work in just the same way as a large impact; force is exerted over a surface area, resulting in pressure. But because these pressure points are so small they aren't individually terribly important; however, taken together all these pressure points create a generalized pressure which is felt on the surface of the material containing the fluid or gas. It's a bit like the corn popping in your microwave or pot: all those bits of corn crashing into one another create pressure which usually results in the lid coming off or the bag (if you have used microwave popcorn) expanding.

CD-ROM activity 8.2

Now, if we consider a fluid at rest, e.g. a glass of water, the pressure within the water is the same no matter which direction you consider. If you take a

single point in the water there will be pressure acting on it from every direction, but not one direction greater than the other; otherwise, the point would be moving. So this means that pressure within static water has no direction, which means it is not a vector quantity. This is called hydrostatic pressure, the pressure of a fluid when it is at rest.

As you will notice in Practical Activity Box 8.2, the deeper a body (e.g. the balloon) is pulled under the water the more crushed it becomes, but we said previously that the pressure was the same

Practical Activity Box 8.2

Blow up a small balloon (not fully); this will represent a single point. Now fill a bucket (a bath would do just as well) with water and immerse the balloon by pulling it under the water at the knot rather than pushing from the top. As you pull the balloon down you will start to find that it reduces in size. This is because of the hydrostatic pressure acting on it, squashing it. Now you should notice that the balloon collapses more at the bottom than at the top (more about this later) and that it is even round the circumference of the balloon; i.e. no one single point is being pushed more than any other at the same depth. This may be difficult to see in your bucket; you could take it to your local swimming pool but that might need some explanation to the lifeguards.

CD-ROM, activity 8.3

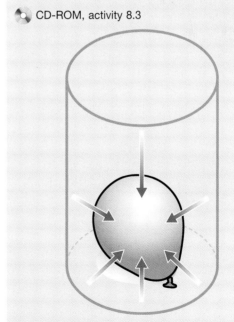

Figure 8.3 • Balloon in a bucket.

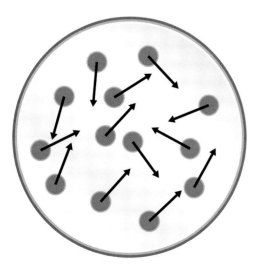

Figure 8.2 • Movement of molecules in gases and fluids.

throughout. Well, it has the same direction throughout but not the same magnitude; pressure in a fluid increases with depth. The weight of the column of water above an immersed point (like your balloon) presses down on the water below; this downward force is simply the mass of the water multiplied by gravity. Now unlike solids; gases and fluids can be compressed (remember when you compressed air in Practical Activity 6.3), which results in an increase in density (more molecules packed together) and therefore more pressure (less space = more collisions = more pressure). This is a bit like when yet another person tries to get into an already packed elevator: less space, more contact among the people (try Practical Activity 8.5). It's the same for the balloon; the increased pressure outside the balloon squeezes the balloon more, which of course its weak rubbery material can't resist and it collapses (see Further Information Box 8.1 on how divers conquered this problem).

Further Information Box 8.1

The increase in hydrostatic pressure with depth has always presented a barrier to deep sea diving (as well as lack of an air supply of course). To prevent the diver being crushed (like the balloon in your bucket) or at the very least find it very difficult to breath, suits were designed as early as the sixteenth century to withstand high pressures. The most important development was making helmets out of hard metal, which protected the brain and eyes and allowed the diver to breathe out.

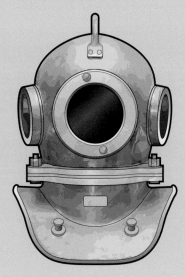

Figure 8.4 • Metal diving helmet.

This relationship between pressure, density and water depth can be expressed by the equation

Hydrostatic pressure = $d \times g \times h$

where d = fluid density, g is gravity and h is the height of the column of water (or depth if you like).

The next couple of activities allow you to explore some properties of fluids, pressure, temperature and volume.

What to remember so far

Density is how closely packed together stuff is. If something is more dense than water it sinks, less and it floats. The human body, on average, just

Practical Activity Box 8.3

When you are next at your local swimming pool stand in the shallow end up to your shoulders. Stay there for 5 minutes, trying not to look suspicious. During this time the higher pressure at your feet compared to your top pushes more blood than normal up into your chest and abdomen, in exactly the same way that air was pushed upwards when you immersed the balloon in the bucket (Practical Activity 8.1). This increased volume of blood centrally can constrict your breathing. You will probably not feel this because it is only a small change but if you had an existing problem with your breathing, being immersed in water may cause you to become short of breath. The increased pressure also increases the rate that your bladder fills (so you need to go to the toilet sooner).

Being immersed in water can have benefits too; e.g. the higher pressure at your feet may help disperse any swelling around your ankle if you had an ankle injury. Perhaps the most obvious benefit of immersion is reduced loading through your joints due to buoyancy (which we will talk about in the next section). This is particularly helpful if you are trying to gradually reintroduce loading through injured parts of the body, e.g. during the rehabilitation of a lower limb fracture. As a rough guideline if you immerse yourself up to:
- Top of shoulders = loading reduced by 90%;
- Bottom of breast bone (sternum) = loading reduced by 66%; and
- Hip bone = loading reduced by 50%.

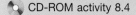 CD-ROM activity 8.4

Practical Activity Box 8.4

Pressure and temperature

Now pressure is also dependent on temperature. Turn the heat up and the molecules move around more, more collisions and therefore more pressure (think of the popcorn). This can be best illustrated with an experiment. Blow up a balloon (if you have any left) and note its size (tape measure or draw round it). Now pop it in the freezer for a couple of hours. When you take it out you will notice that it is much smaller. Put it on a table and watch what happens. The change is all to do with temperature since the amount of air within the balloon has remained the same. At room temperature the air particles are smashing into each other and pressing against the side of the balloon; at low temperatures the particles lose their energy and move less. With nothing pressing against the side of the balloon it collapses.

Practical Activity Box 8.5

Pressure and volume

Blow up a balloon but not to the point of bursting, just reasonably well inflated. What you have done is push a lot of air molecules into the rubber balloon. The pressure from all these molecules moving about is being felt by the walls of the balloon and this internal pressure causes it to expand. Now put your hands around the balloon and squeeze so that the balloon gets smaller (without bursting). The volume (space occupied by the air molecules) reduces so there will be more impacts among the molecules which increases pressure of the walls of the balloon, a pressure you should be feeling.

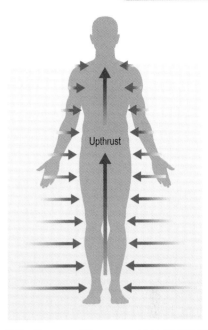

Figure 8.5 • Pressure difference on an immersed body causing upthrust.

about floats. Water pressure increases the deeper you go. If you stand up to your neck in water there will be more pressure at your feet than at your neck (try Practical Activity 8.3). Temperature can also affect pressure: higher temperatures, higher pressure (provided the stuff is contained within the shape) (try Practical Activity 8.4).

Archimedes principle, buoyancy and Pascal's law

The difference in pressure of an immersed object between the top (low pressure) and bottom (high pressure) causes something called upthrust, better known as **buoyancy** (see Fig. 8.5). If you had a long thin balloon and squeezed it more at one end than the other the air moves along to the unsqueezed end, bulging that end out more. It may even jump out of your hand like a bar of soap. This is essentially **Pascal's law** in action: a change in pressure (like you squeezing the balloon) is conveyed to the rest of the gas or fluid and to the surfaces of the container. This also explains buoyancy, which is a force we all know from our times in the swimming pool; this is the force that works against us as we try to touch the bottom of the pool. This is the force that caused Archimedes to leap out of his bath crying 'Eureka!' (see Further Information Box 8.2). On entering his bath Archimedes displaced a certain amount of water; the more he displaced, the greater the upward thrust (buoyancy). This was known as **Archimedes principle** that an object immersed in water creates an upward thrust (buoyancy) equal to the weight of the displaced water. You will have experienced this effect in Practical Activity 8.1: the more of the balloon that was immersed, the greater the force pushing it up. Buoyancy can be very useful in rehabilitation by providing a means of resisting movement as well as supporting painful limbs (see Practical Activity Box 8.3).

Archimedes of Syracuse

Archimedes was a pretty stunning individual in terms of the inventions and discoveries attributed to him. He lived more than 2,000 years ago in a port called Syracuse, which still exists, down at the bottom of Italy. He died aged 75 years during a war with the Romans while, legend has it, trying to protect his scientific instruments. He spent most of his time solving mathematical and engineering problems. Among his inventions was the Archimedes screw, which is a method of transporting water uphill using a pipe with an internal helical winding system which literally scoops up the water. The simplicity and effectiveness of the design has stood the test of time such that it is still used today by farmers in some parts of the world as well as for draining the polders in the Netherlands.

As we have found in this chapter Archimedes also discovered the principle of buoyancy, a discovery inspired by a local ruler's need to measure the quantity of gold in his crown!

Take the pressure off

The way that a contained fluid (or gas) behaves when pressure is applied to it (passing on the change in pressure to the rest of the fluid) provides an effective way of coping with high pressure points. For example, a cushion filled with gel will evenly distribute pressure created at the hip and pelvic bones while seated, a useful characteristic for someone at risk of damage due to prolonged periods of pressure which may disturb blood flow to an area, e.g. bed-bound patients and wheelchair sportsmen. Pascal's law is also the principle underpinning the use of air pockets in the design of running shoes and the introduction of gel pads to the gloves and saddles of cyclists: to distribute pressure evenly, avoiding high points of pressure. This pressure-relieving mechanism is not something that has escaped nature. For example, the fat pads of the heel work in a similar way to distribute pressure when the heel strikes the ground during gait; see Figure 7.3.

Air pressure

Now here is an interesting point and one that might help you interpret the weather report or at least the barometer in your grandfather's house; air, or atmospheric, pressure works in the same way as hydrostatic pressure.

As you sit there reading this book you are being crushed by air above you. Just like the water in the bucket, air increases in density the deeper it gets, being most dense when it is next to the Earth's surface. This is measured by a barometer. So if you go too high up, like in a plane, the density of air might get so low that there aren't enough oxygen molecules around for you. This is why the air inside a plane is pumped to keep the pressure the same as it was (more or less) at ground level.

Now, the difference with hydrostatic pressure was that it was contained, and therefore had the same direction throughout. The difficulty with atmospheric air is that it is not contained, so air pressure might be greater in one direction than in another which causes air to move. So we get areas of high pressure and therefore low pressure and the system attempts, but never succeeds for very long, to reach pressure equilibrium, i.e. the same pressure throughout (see Further Information Box 8.3).

Differences in air pressure are important to sailors. It's one of the factors that create wind (the others being the spinning motion of the Earth and temperature differences which causes convection currents). There is an area around the equator called the Doldrums, which is essentially an area of stable low air pressure caused by the high temperatures. Without a nearby area of high pressure there is very little wind. Consequently sailing ships can be marooned for days or even weeks. This has led to the use of the phrase 'down in the Doldrums' to mean inactivity or even a state of despondency.

Mechanics of flow

We have considered fluids and gases at rest, with all the forces in balance. If there is an unbalanced force, e.g. the heart pumping blood, a fan pushing air, or you squeezing one end of a balloon, then fluids and gases will move. They flow. This movement occurs in layers, one layer of the fluid sliding over the one next to it (this is exactly the same as shear strain; see Practical Activity Box 6.1). This kind of movement in layers is called **laminar flow**; the main factor which affects laminar flow is the stickiness between the layers, which is the same as

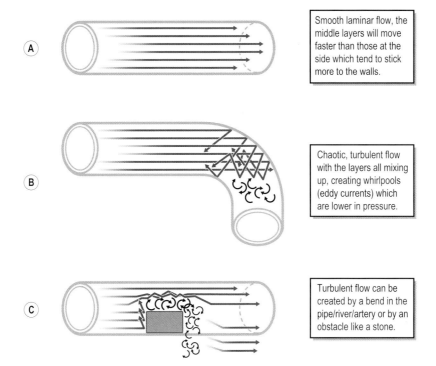

A: Smooth laminar flow, the middle layers will move faster than those at the side which tend to stick more to the walls.

B: Chaotic, turbulent flow with the layers all mixing up, creating whirlpools (eddy currents) which are lower in pressure.

C: Turbulent flow can be created by a bend in the pipe/river/artery or by an obstacle like a stone.

Figure 8.6 • Laminar and turbulent flow.

viscosity (resistant to flow) that we talked about in Chapter 6. So the layers of treacle, for example, will slip over each other more slowly than water. The layers next to the containing surface (artery wall, sides of swimming pool, etc.) will move the slowest. They kind of stick to the sides, whereas the layers in the middle will move fastest. This type of flow is demonstrated in Figure 8.6A.

You can imagine this movement in layers like the lanes of a motorway. The lane on the inside moves slowly with greater movement in the overtaking layers so that the fastest cars travel in the lane closest to the central reservation. Just like the motorway laminar flow continues smoothly until it comes across an obstacle or is forced to make a change in direction. This causes the layers to mix (like cars changing lanes), producing what is called **turbulent flow**; see Figure 8.7.

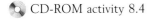 CD-ROM activity 8.4

Drag

The turbulence your hand produced in the bucket or bath (you need to try Practical Activity 8.6 first) is partly responsible for a force that acts in the opposite

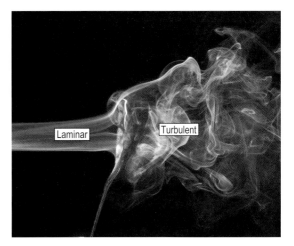

Figure 8.7 • Laminar and turbulent flow from a burning match.

direction to the motion; this force is called **drag**. Drag only occurs when a body (brick, person, bike, plane, bird) travels through a liquid or gas (really what we are talking about here is water and air). So if you are just sitting in the swimming pool you won't experience drag. Drag comes from a couple of different factors. Firstly there is friction between the moving body and the water/air molecules. In this

Practical Activity Box 8.6

Next time it rains heavily take a trip to your nearest river (once the rain has abated) and from a safe vantage point observe the way the river flows. Place a stick into the river close to the bank, and note how fast it moved. This is the slow lane of the river. Now throw another one into the middle; this is the fast lane. If you have ducks inhabiting your river you will notice that they don't swim up the middle of a river; intelligently they use the slow lane to move upstream.

If you haven't got a river close by or it is still raining then try this alternative: Fill your bucket or bath again with lukewarm water; around about 30 cm of depth should do it. Now, unlike the river this is a contained liquid but we can still observe laminar and turbulent flow by moving objects through it, in this case your hand. Place your hand flat in the water and move it sideways, keeping your fingers pointing down as if you were imitating a shark's dorsal fin. The water moves smoothly around your hand, laminar flow. Now turn your hand so that you are pushing the water with the palm of your hand. This time you should see some frothy water and little whirlpools (also known as eddy current) behind your hand. This is the result of turbulent flow, the layers of water mixing with each other. Adjust the speed of your hand. You should find that the faster it gets, the more turbulence is created.

case friction works in exactly the same way as it did on land: the rougher the surface, the greater the coefficient of friction (see Chapter 4). So if you want to reduce drag, make the surface of your body smooth; you don't have to look far to find evidence to support this. Consider the skinsuits worn by competitive swimmers and cyclists, designed with reducing friction in mind. Can you think of another example of something made with its outer surface smooth to reduce friction? When you think about it anything that goes fast is designed in this way: smooth surfaces.

The other main cause of drag is the shape of the body moving through the water/air; this is called **form drag**. Remember in Practical Activity 8.6, there was more turbulence created when you turned your hand round so you were 'pushing' the water with the palm of your hand. Your hand, or any other moving object, is literally pushing the layers apart so that it can occupy the space where the air/water molecules were. The more water there is, the more difficult it is to prise the layers

apart. It's a bit like when you take a walk in the woods at the peak of summer; you have to push apart the overgrown plants obstructing the path you are walking down. The more plants there are, the more difficult this task is. If you are squeezing along an overgrown path you shape your body so that it is narrower at the front; e.g. you may turn sideways. This means you are pushing against less vegetation, and it doesn't have to move as far (so less effort). Moving through water or air is exactly the same. Afterall they both still contain mass which must be pushed aside.

As an object hits the water/air a large front end will mean more water/air is pushed aide (like a very wide person trying to move down your overgrown path). It will also mean the layers of air/water will mix up (see Figures 8.6B, 8.6C and 8.7), causing turbulence. So the trick is to gradually separate the layers of water so they continue to flow in layers over the object. By presenting a narrow front surface which gradually slopes back the layers can flow over the object with minimal disruption. Again this principle is behind the design of many fast-travelling bodies/objects, e.g. the pointed nose cone of a rocket. This principle is also followed in sport; for example, divers enter the swimming pool with their arms stretched out and their head tucked to minimize disruption of the water. They are trying to slip between the layers of water; in fact they are scored on exactly this.

Although bodies and machines have been designed to be more aerodynamic, or hydrodynamic if going through water, they can't completely avoid drag and the worse bit is that the faster they move the greater the drag. No wonder so much design time is spent reducing friction and improving the shape.

Bernoulli's principle

Speed affects drag by something known as **Bernoulli's principle**, which states that pressure will reduce the faster that water or air moves. As you probably noticed when moving your hand through the bucket (Practical Activity 8.6), the turbulence created is behind the moving object. Move it fast enough and you will probably see eddy currents (Figure 8.6B, C). Because the water is moving much faster when it is turbulent the pressure decreases. This drop in pressure pulls (perhaps sucks is a better word) the body backwards.

Again this is something you will be aware of in everyday life and especially with things that move

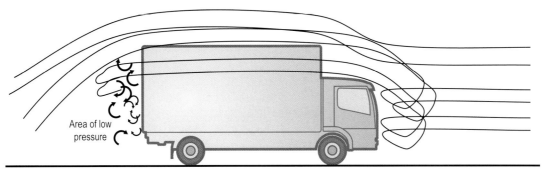

Figure 8.8 • Turbulent flow behind a moving lorry creating an area of low pressure; Bernoulli's principle.

fast. Imagine yourself walking along a pavement and a large lorry whisks past you. Depending on the speed and size of the lorry you will experience some sensation of being pulled into the back of lorry, sometimes people refer to this as the wake or slip stream. The reason for the pulling sensation is this area of low pressure immediately behind the lorry caused by the fast moving turbulent air (Fig. 8.8).

Another example of this can be observed in the spring time at your local river/pond. At this time of year you might observe a train of ducklings flowing along in the water behind their mother. They aren't really as fast as their mother; they are just using this sucking effect of the fast-flowing water to help them keep up. Being pulled along in your parents' wake is probably quite an enjoyable experience, that is, until the day you decide to move off in a different direction.

Drag is usually described as a horizontal force, pulling on an object which is moving forwards (or backwards) through air/water. However, it can also act vertically; the wings of a plane are shaped so that the air flows faster above the wing than below. As you now know this creates a low pressure above the wing which the aircraft is sucked into. This is the same as drag but when it acts perpendicularly (at right angles) to the motion it is called lift. Now that you know a little about aerodynamics why not have a go at Practical Activity 8.7.

Blood flow: haemodynamics

As we are dealing with the human body, when we talk about flow we need to talk about the main thing that flows around our body: blood. Blood is more viscous than water, so it tends to move that bit slower. Well it would if it didn't have a pump (your heart) which periodically (once every second or so)

Practical Activity Box 8.7

Aerodynamics and cycling

Next time the Tour de France (or any other bicycle race) is on the television make a note to watch it. Professional cyclists put into place all the principles of aerodynamics. See if you can observe any of the following:

1. Smooth skin-hugging clothes;
2. Bikes smoothed with the joints in the frame rounded;
3. Low riding position, back flat and body crouched over the handle bars;
4. A back wheel that is filled in with a disk;
5. Helmets shaped like a teardrop at the back;
6. Riders cycling very closely behind each other; and
7. Shaved legs.

Now identify from the following list what the riders are trying to achieve with each of these strategies:

a. Reduce friction;
b. Reduce form drag; or
c. Take advantage of negative pressure.

Answers are in Appendix 8.

increases the pressure. Blood flow through arteries behaves the same way as other liquids: laminar flow until obstacles are met, the artery narrows or there is a change in direction, e.g. moving around bent joints. This will create turbulence, which, as we now know, lowers pressure. Too much turbulence therefore means you need to turn up the pump to keep the same blood pressure. So if you want to keep turbulence to a minimum you will need to keep all your joints straight, which is clearly not practical.

Fast-flowing turbulent blood may also lead to specific sites of arterial inflammation due to damage to the endothelium wall of the artery with longer-term consequences of scar tissue. This area of bio-mechanics is still developing and we may yet get more understanding of musculoskeletal pain through altered haemodynamics.

Further Information Box 8.4

Flow was well understood by the ancient Egyptians. Life depended on controlling the water flow from the Nile through the basic, but effective irrigation and damming system which still sustains a huge population. Transport along the Nile during the time of the Pharaohs was also so much easier if you understood air flow so that you effectively positioned the sails on your felucca (Egyptian sailing boat).

Finally the Egyptians had an understanding, albeit grisly, of body fluids. The process of mummification involves the draining of body fluids into jars. The fact that Egyptians understood this took time and could be helped by gravity conjures up a pretty grisly image.

What you need to remember from all that

Objects float or sink in gas or liquid depending on their relative density. The pressure within a static liquid has the same direction throughout but will increase with depth. Pressure can be altered by volume and temperature. Pressure differences within a liquid cause upthrust (buoyancy), which can be used by therapists. Pressure within a liquid is evened out, which is called Bernoulli's principle and can be used to reduce specific areas of high pressure. Pressure differences within gases and liquids cause movement which tends to be in layers (laminar) but can become turbulent (layers mix) if flow is rapid or an obstruction is met. Turbulent flow causes areas of low pressure, which is one of the factors behind drag (a force opposing forward motion), the other being friction.

Chapter Nine

Energy and Movement

What you will learn about in this chapter

1. What energy is;
2. Different forms of energy;
3. Movement strategies to optimize energy consumption; and
4. Measuring the energy of movement.

Words you will come across

Potential energy, kinetic energy, elastic energy.

What energy is

Evolution has fine-tuned us over millennia to be the most physically versatile creatures on Earth. In many ways movement defines us individually and provides the necessary foundation for intellectual development. The way we walk, the hand gestures we use when we talk and the way we hold a cup are expressions of our style and personality.

Even though we have many individual movement mannerisms that help express our individual character we all, more or less, move in the same way. The predictability of many movements has allowed movement scientists to study and characterize the key elements of movements such as walking, standing up from a chair and reaching for a cup. This has ultimately led to a better understanding, and therefore management, of movement disorders

such as cerebral palsy and Parkinson's disease. Sports professionals also use greater understanding of movement to improve sports performance as well as to reduce risks of injury.

There are three good reasons for movement patterns being similar:

1. **Anatomy:** We all (more or less) have the same basic body shape and parts.

2. **Environment:** We all must function in a common environment, so things like chair height, cup size, height of a tennis net are the same for everyone. To some degree clothes can also be considered an environmental factor that shapes our movement.

3. **Energy economics**: We are all driven by the same desire to minimize the energy cost of movement. Our natural inclination is to conserve energy.

To a lesser extent culture and even mood shape our movement patterns; this may be the swaggering gait of a cabaret singer or the slow careful steps of a philosopher deep in thought.

It is beyond the scope of this book to discuss the first two reasons for movement pattern, nevermind the influence of culture or mood on movement, interesting though these aspects are. The third reason, 'energy conservation', will be explored in this chapter. But first we need to clarify what we mean by energy. Although this was covered in Chapter 5 it is worth defining, because it is a critical concept and one that will give you greater depth to understanding human movement.

Potential and kinetic energy

In mechanical terms energy is the ability of a body to perform work; it exists in two main forms, potential and kinetic energy.

Potential energy

Potential energy depends on the body's position. So a ball sitting on a table has potential energy due to its height; it has the potential to do some work. If you took the table away it would travel toward the ground. If you attached a pulley and some string, it could pull an object along the table. The driving force here is gravity see (see Fig. 9.1).

The potential energy (E_p) an object has due to gravity can be calculated simply as:

**E_p = mass (of body) × gravity (9.81 m/s/s)
    × height (metres)**

and is measured in joules (see Further Information Box 5.1).

So a man weighing 70 kg and standing on a diving board 10 m above the water has

**E_p = 70 × 9.81 × 10
    = 6867 J**

It doesn't have to depend on gravity. Anything which, in its current position, has the potential to perform work has potential energy so a stone placed on a catapult and pulled back has potential energy. A ball filled with air placed at the bottom of a swimming pool has the potential to perform work. If you released the ball it would rise to the top and probably lift into the air. If you released the catapult the stone would fly rapidly towards its target.

Kinetic energy

Kinetic energy is the capacity a body has to work due to its motion. Any moving object has kinetic energy. Imagine a golf club swinging towards a ball. Without consideration to technique the faster the club is moving, the greater capacity it has to do work on the ball (move it forwards and up). Mass is again an important consideration. A heavier club travelling faster has greater capacity to move the ball than a light one. The actual calculation for kinetic energy (E_k) is

$E_k = \frac{1}{2}$ mass × (velocity^2)

see Further Information Box 9.1 for difference between kinetic energy and momentum.

A body will move between potential and kinetic energy states. While moving it may be gaining potential energy and as it loses potential energy it may be gaining kinetic energy. Imagine a cyclist on top of a hill, he has potential energy due to his height above the ground (just like the ball on top of the table) as he speeds down the hill he loses height and therefore potential energy but will be gaining velocity i.e. kinetic energy, as well as heat

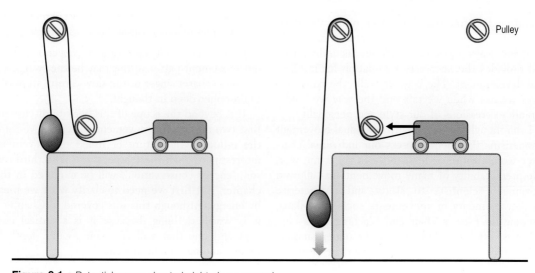

Figure 9.1 • Potential energy due to height above ground.

Further Information Box 9.1

Kinetic energy and momentum

You may recall (Chapter 4, p. 49) that momentum was the product of mass and velocity (mass × velocity), which makes it seem quite similar to kinetic energy (½ mass × (velocity²)). But, because velocity is squared when calculating kinetic energy, an increase in velocity will increase the body's kinetic energy more than its momentum. Although they are both measures of the physical nature of a body in motion there are some differences besides their calculations and SI units. Kinetic energy (in fact all energy) is a scalar quantity; it has no direction. Momentum on the other hand is a vector so it needs a direction. An illustration of this distinction is in the collision between two bodies. Let's imagine two pizza chefs standing at either end of a restaurant throwing balls of dough at each other so that the balls collide, stick together and come to a stop in the middle of the restaurant. Before the collision each dough ball had momentum (mass × velocity). However, because they are in opposite directions this momentum cancels out so that the combined dough ball has a momentum of 0 before and therefore after.

For example, dough ball A has a mass of 1 kg and a velocity of 5 m/s directed from front door to back door (momentum of 5 kg/m/s) and dough ball B has a mass of 2 kg and a velocity of 2.5 m/s directed

from back door to front door (momentum of −5 kg/m/s; I have decided that this direction is negative). So total before collision would be 0 (+5 kg/m/s and −5 kg/m/s = 0). Therefore total momentum after collision would be 0. If the momentum before was not 0 then after the collision the ball would have some momentum. But what about kinetic energy? Before the collision dough ball A has 12.5 J of kinetic energy and dough ball B has 6.25 J. Energy is a scalar so no negatives; therefore the total energy before collision was 18.75 J (12.5 J + 6.25 J = 18.75 J). The collision caused the dough balls to stop moving (they stuck together—no kinetic energy), so kinetic energy, unlike momentum, is not conserved. No movement. Energy, however, is not lost. Instead it is converted to other energy forms; e.g. the dough balls will have a higher temperature (thermal energy, which is really another form of kinetic energy but let's not get too microscopic here).

So momentum and kinetic energy are clearly related but not equivalent. Momentum is always conserved when bodies come in contact with each other (the net momentum is always the same), whereas kinetic energy can increase and decrease, through conversion into other forms of energy; importantly the total amount of energy (in all its states) is always conserved.

---

if the brakes are applied (heat will also occur due to friction between the road and tyre). As the next hill approaches this kinetic energy is converted to potential, you gain height but the bike slows down. At the top of the hill potential energy is restored, ready for another speedy descent.

CD-ROM activity 9.1

One of the fundamental laws of nature is that energy cannot be destroyed or created. But as we have seen it can flow from one form to another. During human movement there is a continual exchange between potential and kinetic energy (see Fig. 9.2).

CD-ROM activity 9.2

The analogy of the cyclists exchanging E_p and E_k can also be used during walking. At mid-stance (one foot swinging past the other) the centre of mass is at its highest (like the cyclists on top of the hill). This is converted to kinetic energy as we 'fall' forwards and down.

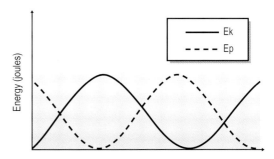

Figure 9.2 • Flow of energy between kinetic and potential states during walking.

Have you ever seen a child drawing a line along a wall with chalk or a stick while they are walking? If you had, you may have noticed that they leave a wavy line behind. This is not artistic creativity on the child's part but rather a consequence of the body rising and falling during walking. It's this very motion that allows pedometers to count your steps; each lift up counts as one step.

Let's go through the walking or gait cycle together and you will hopefully see what I mean. There is a tutorial on the gait cycle in your CD-ROM which will help you with the phases and events.

First of all stand up, at this point your centre of mass (CoM) is at its highest (55% of your height; see p. 19). Now take a step forwards. As you do your CoM will fall (both legs are at an angle) by around 5 cm. This fall is just the same as the cyclist speeding down the hill, potential energy converted to kinetic. Of course your body continues to move (kinetic energy) and this energy is used to help the body lift up again to the height you were while standing at the start (highest point). Once at the top again your body has regained the potential energy ready for another fall (see Fig. 9.3). This swinging pendulum model of walking has been suggested to be very efficient, as it uses existing energy in the body to keep the body moving, so efficient that scientists have tried to recreate this in models called passive walkers—see Further Information Box 9.2.

Elastically stored potential energy

As we discussed previously in Chapter 6 potential energy can be stored in a piece of stretched elastic material. The energy used to stretch open a spring or rubber band will be returned immediately when it returns, on release, to its original shape. We explored this a little in Chapter 6 with the compression of a ball on impact with the ground or air

> ### Further Information Box 9.2
>
> Scientists have tried for a long time to perfect models of walking that use minimal energy. This invariably means using some kind of pendulum swing to keep the model moving forwards. So the walking commences with someone lifting the pendulum up, the release of the pendulum providing the initial power to the walker to take a series of steps through a series of friction-free hinges (see Fig. 9.4 for an example). This is just like an obliging parent pulling back the swing with their child in it. Releasing the swing commences the cycling pendulum motion of the swing.
>
> Inevitably, without any further pushing, the child's swing slows down and, despite a lot of tinkering, this also happens to the passive walking models. This has meant that these models still need some kind of energy input (like the parent giving the swing a little push now and again); usually this is provided by getting the model to walk down a slope, so the energy comes from gravity.

being compressed in a bicycle pump. Nature has incorporated this method of storing energy by developing the elastic properties of connective tissue and tendons in particular; see Further Information Box 9.3 for a really interesting example. There are also more details on the elastic properties of tissue in Chapters 6 and 7.

Shortening a muscle is quite an inefficient, energy-expensive action, so the body tries to minimize this whenever possible. Fortunately we have connective

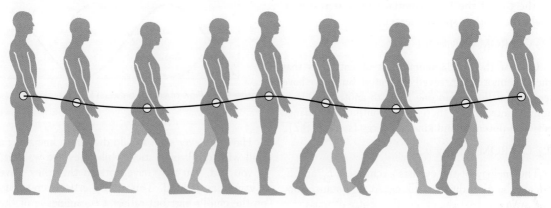

First step: Both feet on ground: Next step lifts   The cycle repeats
CoM lowers   CoM at lowest   CoM again

Figure 9.3 • Vertical displacement of centre of mass during gait.

Further Information Box 9.3

The Achilles tendon appears to have developed as a consequence of bipedal upright walking and running. Rather than a weak spot as the unfortunate story of the hero of Greek mythology 'Achilles' tells us, the development of the Achilles tendon is a key evolutionary step. The absence of similarly well-developed Achilles tendons in other primates is a refection of its importance to human upright gait.

Researchers at Manchester University created a simulation from the fossilized remains of the earliest walking hominid—Lucy—and found the evolution of the Achilles tendon was an important step (excuse the pun) in the development of efficient walking and running. They estimated the tendon probably developed between two and three and half million years ago.

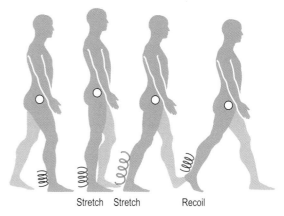

Stretch   Stretch   Recoil

Figure 9.5 • Storing elastic energy in the calf muscles to assist forward movement of the leg when walking.

tissue in our muscle (tendons and muscle harness—see Chapter 8) which can act as passive springs (no active work) to store kinetic energy during movement; this is a very efficient strategy. This is what the body tries to utilize when walking, a strategy so efficient that the elastic recoil of the Achilles tendon has been estimated to contribute up to 60% of the energy required for normal walking. But how does it do this? Let's have a look at how this happens by looking at the stance phase of gait. In Figure 9.5 just consider the darkened side, which is the leg that stays on the ground, otherwise known as the stance leg.

At the start of the sequence (gait cycle) the forward rotation of the tibia over a foot planted firmly on the ground basically winds up the Achilles tendon (and other elastic components of the calf) like a spring. As the body continues to rotate forwards the spring is released which helps to push the body up and forwards.

Elastic storage is not just a strategy used during gait; it contributes to other movements. Let's consider the sit-to-stand movement. The initial part of the sit-to-stand movement involves the individual flexing their head, arms and trunk forward. What does this do to the hamstring muscles? Best way to find out is to try it yourself. While sitting place both your hands under your thighs and lean forwards reasonably quickly, as if you were about to stand up.

CD-ROM activity 9.3, video clips of the sit to stand movement.

What you felt (I hope) was an eccentric contraction (see p. 9). The muscle is active (tensing under your hand) while lengthening (the hamstrings attach to the pelvis which is moving forwards, lengthening the muscle). This eccentric contraction controls the forward movement of the trunk but it also helps the muscle to store elastic energy (see Fig. 9.6). The added tension within the muscle due to contraction makes the 'muscle spring' even stiffer, and, as I am sure you know, if you can stretch out a stiff spring it will spring back with more force than a slack one.

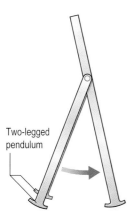

Two-legged pendulum

There are two pendulums in this passive walker. One of the pendulums has two points of contact with the ground (two legs) and the other has only one, this is to improves it's stability. At the point shown the walker is very stable (all feet on the ground) however the two-legged pendulum is about to advance over the single-legged pendulum (which will act like an inverted pendulum) driven by the force of gravity.

Figure 9.4 • Example of passive walking model.

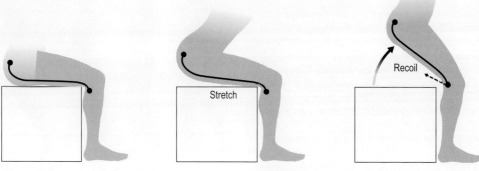

Figure 9.6 • Using elastic storage during the sit to stand movement.

So, if you stretch a muscle while it is under tension it will release with even greater force. If this recoil is timed with a concentric contraction the muscle will be able to create very large forces indeed (try Practical Activity 9.2).

This behaviour of muscle is known in the sports world as the stretch shortening cycle (SSC). It has been well studied in animals and turkeys in particular which, due to their proportionally large amounts of tendon, are pretty efficient runners.

Practical Activity Box 9.1

Can you observe the stretch shortening cycle in other movements or in other muscle groups? Look at the way someone performs a vertical jump or the muscle activity during the triple jump. What about a javelin throw? Are there other muscle groups using SSC during gait apart from the calf muscles?

Sports coaches and physiotherapists design exercise programmes to train this property of skeletal muscle. Plyometric exercises start with a stretching phase consisting of an eccentric contraction immediately followed by a rapid concentric contraction. The classic example of this is jumping down from a step. Upon landing the extensor muscles of the lower limb (muscles that straighten the hip, knee and ankle) are stretched and eccentrically contract. This action is immediately followed by a powerful extension of the same muscles to accelerate the body up. Repetitions of this activity are said to train the elastic recoil ability of these muscles, which is useful in sports that include explosive movements such as volleyball and the high jump.

Practical Activity Box 9.2

Hold the thumb of your right hand with the thumb and index finger of your left. Now stretch it down towards your forearm (see Fig. 9.7). You probably won't be able to make it touch your forearm but just bring it down enough so that you can feel a stretch on the back of your wrist. Let go.

The spring back of your thumb comes from elastic energy stored in your connective tissue. Now do the same thing but this time push a little against your thumb being stretched down (basically try to resist the stretch a little). This time when you let go you should have found your thumb/wrist bounced back further and faster, an illustration of the added effect an eccentric contraction can have on elastic recoil.

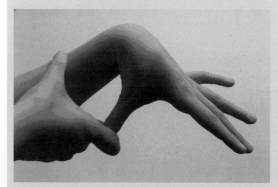

Figure 9.7 • Practical activity 9.2

Energy conservation

The word conservation implies there is something to lose but we know that energy cannot be created or destroyed. So what we mean by conservation is really a loss of energy that is useful to the task, so the heat given off by a car engine doesn't really help the car move forward (just provides a nice warm surface for cats, once parked).

Mechanical engineers and scientists have long strived for a machine or system of machines that conserve their energy in the single useful form. The perpetual motion machine was an engineer's holy grail for many centuries, leading to pretty amazing machines (see Further Information Box 5.5). However, in practice these machines could not exist since there is always some energy exchange to heat or light through friction or air resistance.

This idea of systems attempting to minimize the loss to other energy forms was behind the explanation of human gait proposed by Inman and Saunders more than 30 years ago. The basic premise of this theory of walking efficiency was that the body minimized movements not directly involved in the forward translation of the body, i.e. to minimize the movement of the body's CoM. They considered up and down and side-to-side movements to be inefficient, since they were not in the direction of travel. So they thought, what does the body do to reduce these movements?

They explored this idea through thought experiments (as opposed to experimental testing): what if there were no joints in the lower limb apart from the hip and that this worked like a simple hinge? This was described as a caliper gait, like opening and closing a pair of scissors.

This model of gait appeared highly inefficient, with the body moving a lot to the side as well as up and down. Why not try it yourself? Obviously you can't get rid of your pelvis, knees and ankles but you could try to keep your knee straight and your ankle in neutral (the way it is when you stand normally). It is quite difficult to walk this way but if you managed you might have noticed a lot more swaying, up and down and side to side, mainly because it is difficult to swing your straight leg through.

This provided Inman and Saunders with a basis for explaining the movements of the lower limb in what became called the **determinants of gait**. They proposed six movements of the lower limb that made walking more efficient, of which we will discuss two.

Stance phase: knee flexion

During the stance phase there is a slight flexion of the knee. This keeps the body low, minimizing the up and down movement. Have a look at the video clip (CD-ROM activity 9.4) from the side and see if you can see the slight knee flexion during mid-stance (when the swinging leg is passing the standing leg).

CD-ROM activity 9.4, clips of the gait cycle from the side

Pelvic list

As the foot impacts with the ground the pelvis lists (drops) downwards on the opposite side. This, it was proposed, minimizes the vertical movement of the body. The best way to think abut this one is to consider what would happen if your pelvis didn't drop. Try it: walk about with your hands on your pelvis (slide your hands down the side of your trunk until you get to the bones—iliac crests). You should feel the pelvis lift and drop in time with the feet striking and then pushing off from the ground. Now just focus on initial contact, and try to keep your pelvis up (don't let it drop down). The effect, as I hope you find, is your body remains higher and shifted out to the side.

CD-ROM activity 9.5, clips of the gait cycle from the front

The advent of sophisticated motion analysis systems has allowed these determinants to be tested under laboratory conditions. It appears that most of them have little impact on the vertical and lateral movement of the body's CoM. In fact the one thing that prevents excessive vertical displacement of the CoM is lifting your heel off the ground at the end of stance phase, a movement which limits the amount of drop your body goes through at the end of stance. Again the best way to demonstrate how this works is by trying it out. As you take a step forward your heel will lift off the ground on the opposite side; now try to keep your heel on the ground. What happens to your body?

This greater drop of your body is not a good idea because now you have to lift it up again at the next step. And what makes your heel come off the ground? Well it is at least helped by elastic recoil of the Achilles tendon.

OK, so if, as I stated at the start of this chapter, our movements are shaped by the need to conserve energy and the determinants of gait fail to contribute a lot to energy efficiency then what mechanisms do we use to limit the energy cost of walking? Well you already have the answers. Firstly we use the energy-efficient pendular motion of the swinging leg and inverted pendulum during stance phase (body pivoting over the fixed foot) just like the passive walkers (see Fig. 9.4). These motions are assisted by 'muscle springs', the Achilles tendon being a good example of this, which release elastic energy created during the motion and stored with the connective tissue (tendon mainly). Despite these efficient body tissues and movement strategies we still need active tension to be generated in the muscles. The muscles transfer kinetic energy to the bones via the tendons but where does the muscle get the energy from?

Muscle energy

Muscle creates tension through the attachment, pull and then release of one protein filament (myosin) on another (actin), which are positioned next to each other. Rather like a group of people grabbing a rope, pulling it, releasing it and then grabbing the next bit along, but done at slightly different times so that the rope doesn't drop. The point is the rope becomes tense with the pull.

The release of calcium within the muscle, triggered by the nerve impulse, exposes a binding site on actin (like a hole), which the myosin protein quickly attaches to (they naturally attract to each other), forming a cross bridge. During this strong connection the myosin rotates, which causes the actin to move. In the presence of a molecule called adenosine triphosphate (ATP), the myosin releases its grasp, ready for the whole process to start again, and in the process alters ATP to adenosine diphosphate (ADP) through the loss of a phosphate (so two phosphates instead of three). So, the natural affinity between the actin and myosin protein filaments is used to create tension with, ATP breaking it up so that another connection can be made. Without ATP the myosin head would be permanently bound to the actin: not very useful.

The ATP molecule is really the energy source within the body, with potential energy bound up in its chemical bonds. It provides energy when it changes from ATP to ADP but needs energy to rebind with its phosphate to make ATP. In this way it is a bit like a rechargeable battery, powering the sliding motion of the muscle filaments as well as providing the energy for other processes within the body. However, like a rechargeable battery it needs an energy source itself to charge up. The source that

provides this energy is of course food. The consumption of 2000 kcal per day is required to provide the necessary energy and raw materials to make the billions and billions of ATP molecules we use and recycle every minute.

Measuring energy during movement

This chapter has considered energy, and how the body has developed strategies and evolved the material it is constructed from to be as energy efficient as possible. This has led many people to consider that the best way to look at movement is not to focus on the individual movements or muscle action but to measure how much energy is being used. When you think about it there is a lot of logic in this way of thinking. Afterall does it really matter how much your arms swing when you walk or which part of your foot strikes the ground first when you run, as long as what you do is efficient for you? Of course there are other things to consider such as stress on different parts of the body but analysing the overall energy cost of a movement can provide really good insight into a movement. So how can this be done?

Well, the best way to do it is directly. The creation of ATP molecules from food (the glucose and fatty acids) requires oxygen (O_2), which is why you need to keep breathing all the time! The more muscles work, the greater creation of ATP, the more O_2 is required. So if you measure how much oxygen you 'consume' during a movement you'll get a pretty good direct measurement of how much energy the movement costs you. Traditionally this was done by collecting the air you have expired in a big bag called a Douglas bag. The collected air was examined to see (a) what volume of air you consumed and (b) how much O_2 you extracted from that air. This technique allowed detailed energy analysis of many different movements (see Table 9.1) but was always felt to encumber the subject by having them carry a bag and have a mask over their face. There have been advances on this technique which have negated the need to collect the gases in a bag. However, you still need to wear a mask.

The delivery of O_2 and nutrients to the muscle depends on blood supply so when more ATP is required for muscle action more blood (carrying O_2

Table 9.1 Energy values for different activities

Population	Activity	Energy cost (kcal/min)
Children	Sitting	0.5
Healthy adults	Watching TV	0.75–1
Healthy adult men	Vacuuming	3.4
Healthy adults	Walking	3
Healthy adults	Cycling	4.4
Healthy adult men	Digging	6.4
Adults with hip problems	Walking	49

These are values approximated from the literature.

and nutrients) is pumped to the muscles. Heart rate is therefore an indirect measurement of the energy cost of a movement. In fact this relationship has been shown to be linear; i.e. as energy cost (measured by O_2 consumption) rises, heart rate goes up by a similar amount. This is good news for those of you working in clinical and sports environments without high-tech equipment. You can get a pretty good estimate of the energy cost of a movement by recording the change in heart rate, i.e. difference between heart rate before commencing activity (at rest) and heart rate during the activity (once a steady rhythm has been established). This relationship does not always hold true when exercising heavily or with people who have problems with their heart which may require drugs to control their heart rate.

What do you need to remember from all that

This chapter covered human movement from the perspective of energy. We looked at what energy was, considering its two basic forms, potential and kinetic energy. We examined how the body fluctuates between potential and kinetic energy and how it makes use of elegant strategies (usually involving pendulums) and elasticity of 'muscle springs' to be as energy efficient as possible during movements, gait and sit-to-stand being offered as examples. Finally we looked at the direct cost of muscle contraction, how energy is supplied to muscles using ATP as a rechargeable battery and how we can measure the energy cost of movement.

Chapter Ten

10

Therapeutic Application of Force

What you will learn about in this chapter

1. Forces applied when mobilizing joints and stretching tissue;
2. The use of drag and buoyancy in hydrotherapy;
3. The use of turbulence and shear force in breathing techniques; and
4. The use of orthotics to alter force direction and distribution.

Techniques considered

Posteroanterior spinal mobilization, massage, static stretch, forced expiratory technique, Halliwick approach to swimming, medial heel wedge, dynamic wrist splinting.

This chapter is concerned with the way therapists in sport and rehabilitation apply and manipulate forces to the body as part of their treatment. It is intended to make you think more about what you are doing when applying forces to the human body and every profession does it, as a matter of course. To mobilize a stiff part of the spine a physiotherapist or osteopath might apply direct downward pressure onto a specific segment. An occupational therapist might construct a hand splint to gradually stretch the tissues overlying a joint to improve function. A shortened hamstring muscle of an athlete might improve from the application of tensile stress by a sports therapist. Let's not forget the podiatrist that designs an insole for a shoe to alter the direction and distribution of forces acting on the foot, knee and hip.

What we'll do is pick some of these techniques, describe them a bit and then take a biomechanical perspective on what it is going on.

Mobilization techniques

The practice of applying force directly to a joint is widely used by many health professionals such as chiropractors, osteopaths and physiotherapists. Interestingly the manner in which these professionals apply this force (magnitude, frequency, rate and direction) can be quite different, and for good biomechanical reasons, which we will touch on later.

Let's look at one specific mobilization technique: a posteroanterior mobilization on the spine (or PA for short). This is a downward force applied to the spinous process of a prone patient (lying on their front). The reason for applying this kind of technique might be to improve the range of motion, in the same way that you might wiggle and jiggle a stiff link in a chain or loosen an old door hinge by opening and shutting it. Some therapists perform the technique to create a sedative effect on the painful segment. Whatever the reason let's look at some of the biomechanical considerations during a typical setup of a therapist applying a PA.

To perform the PA the therapist stands at the side of the patient who is lying on their front on a plinth (firm bed) and applies downward pressure at the stiff segment (Fig. 10.1). The magnitude of this downward force is hard for the therapist to measure exactly but using strain gauges (see Chapter 3) values between 63 and 347 N (quite a difference!) have

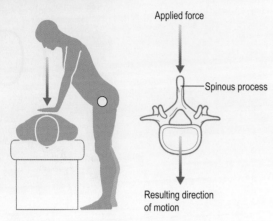

Applied force

Spinous process

Resulting direction
of motion

Figure 10.1 • A physiotherapist applying a PA mobilization
to the lumbar spine, typical direction of applied force.

been recorded, although it should be said that anything between 100 and 150 N seems to be typical, equivalent to 10–15 bags of sugar (see Further Information Box 10.1). The force can be applied through the thumbs of the therapist (surface area approximately 15 cm^2) onto the skin lying over the spinous process. This creates pressure on the skin of around 666 N/cm^2, making it quite uncomfortable for the therapist and patient. For this reason some therapists will use the larger surface area of the hypothenar eminence (pad of soft tissue in the hand just beyond the wrist crease on the little finger side). This compressive stress is applied cyclically (on/off/on/off etc.) at a rate of around 5 times per second, or 5 Hz.

Although this is quite a lot of pressure it is unlikely to strain any of the underlying soft tissues (skin, fat, muscle, blood vessels and nerves) beyond their elastic limits. So when the pressure is released the tissues will quickly reform. If the tissues are only mildly strained what is the point in this mobilizing technique? If you recall from Chapters 6 and 7 the purpose of repetitive force application may not be to actually change the length of tissues or displace the underlying joint but rather to unstiffen the tissues surrounding the joint(s) by altering their viscosity. This ability of connective tissue to become more fluid (less viscous) with repetitive loading is called thixotropy (see p. 86). So it's the repetitive nature of the technique, and not necessarily the magnitude of the force that's important. But what about the underlying bone and joint, which, afterall, is the target of the technique, to cause one segment to move on the one next to it, i.e. to move the joint?

Bone is a much stiffer material than the surrounding soft tissues, which strain. So when the downward

force is applied, the bone (and consequently the joint) will hopefully move because it acts like a rigid body (doesn't change shape). It's a little like pushing an armchair across a carpet to get a better view of the TV. Initially your push squashes (compresses) the chair's soft cushioning; after this your push begins to move the much stiffer frame of the chair. However, unlike other joints (and armchairs) segments of the spine are very closely bound together through bony congruency, joint capsules, large discs, strong ligaments and multiple layers of muscle. So it behaves more like a beam than individual segments (see Fig. 6.9 for a reminder on how a beam strains and try Practical Activity 10.1).

Practical Activity Box 10.1

You will need a few friends for this activity; five or six should do it. Get your friends to stand up in a line and link arms so that they are holding each other really tightly. Now go up to one of your friends in the middle of this human chain and push them. What happened?

This is similar to what happens to your spine when you push one segment: of course the whole chain moves. This means that the side of the spine/human chain you are pressing on will come close together (compressive strain) and the back of the chain will be opened apart (tensile strain).

CD-ROM activity 10.1, video of spine bending

Like the bending force applied at a beam there will be tensile stress on the lower part of the spine and compressive stress on the upper part (see Fig. 10.2). The magnitude of force applied in a PA (100–150 N) is unlikely, after it has been partially reduced by straining the soft tissues, to cause a great deal of displacement. Two to 8 mm has been estimated from mathematical models.

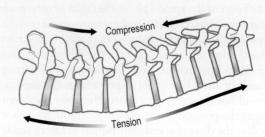

Compression

Tension

Figure 10.2 • Bending stress.

Let's change the setup for this mobilizing force and see what happens. We will ask the therapist to take a small step backwards. This is an easy alteration to make when applying the technique but does it change the effect in any way?

If you remember the principles of force resolution (Chapter 3) you will know that because this force is being applied at an angle, it resolves into components at right angles to each other. So some of the force will still be directed vertically down (but with a reduced magnitude) to produce the same vertically directed motion as before. However, some of the force will now be directed horizontally along the surface of the body (as indicated in Fig. 10.3).

The effect of this horizontal component would be to generate an anticlockwise moment on the vertebra (as shown in Fig. 10.3) because it is applied at a distance from the fulcrum (which in this case is the centre of mass of the vertebra). However, this moment depends on the tissues overlying the spinous process being rigid enough to translate the force. To let you understand what I mean try Practical Activity 10.2.

So you can see that a force applied to the spinous process at an angle is a very different proposition from one applied directly down: different direction, different point of application (if the soft tissues slide) and different magnitude. A small step backwards can dramatically change the technique.

In this mobilization technique we have considered the direction of the force, the point of application, the effect of overlying soft tissues and the repetitive loading but we haven't thought about rate of application, how quickly or slowly the force is applied. In Chapters 6 and 7 we discovered that tissue behaves differently if you apply the force at different rates. So a slow force application allows connective tissue to flow, producing a change in length (without damage), whereas a rapid application causes the tissues to behave more stiffly, which means that the point when plastic changes occur (i.e. tissue became damaged) is reached earlier (you may recall the tearing activity on p. 85).

Practical Activity Box 10.2

Press down on this page with one finger and angle it towards the middle (you may have to hold the book steady) so that the page buckles. Did you find that difficult? Did your finger keep slipping? Now lick the end of your finger and try again. This should prove easier to do because the moisture effectively stuck your finger to the page (increased the coefficient of friction). This time when you pushed the page (hopefully) it moved but it was probably only the top page. This is because there is not much friction between the layers or pages. The same is true for the layers of tissue under the top surface of skin in your own body.

Find a bit of your skin, e.g. the back of your hand, inside of your elbow, etc., and press directly down on the skin with your finger. Now (without changing the force of your press) turn your finger so it is now pressing on your skin at an angle. You should find that your finger (a) isn't pressing down as much and (b) moves over your skin because the layers of soft tissue are sliding on each other. So when applied at an angle the strain becomes more shear than compressive.

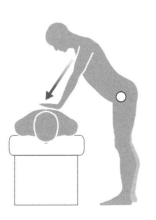
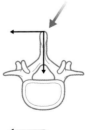

Because the force is applied at an angle there will be force and therefore motion in different directions as shown.

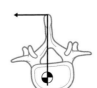

The horizontal component of the force will now cause an anti-clockwise moment because its point of application is a distance from the fulcrum.

Figure 10.3 • A physiotherapist applying a PA mobilization to the lumbar spine, changing the direction of applied force.

A rapidly applied mobilization technique (sometimes referred to as a manipulation) is more likely to damage the connective tissue, but this may be exactly what the practitioner is trying to achieve; perhaps by breaking constraining tissue the joint becomes more mobile. So there are many biomechanical variables to consider when applying a PA. Understanding them will make your technique more effective.

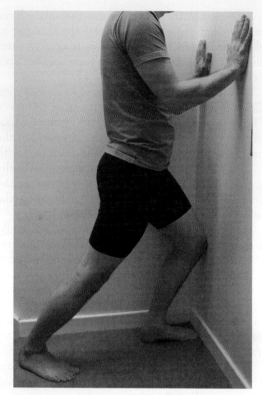

Figure 10.4 • Static stretching of the gastrocnemius (calf) muscle, ankle dorsiflexed and knee straight.

Further Information Box 10.1

In an effort to understand, as well as standardize, spinal mobilizations, simulators are becoming increasingly popular in universities and training institutes. These vary but usually include a mocked-up spine complete with the overlying soft tissues and some way of measuring force such as a strain gauge (see p. 41). The novice practitioner now has the ability to practice their technique while receiving information on direction, rate, frequency, magnitude and point of application of their force. They may for example be able to compare themselves to an experienced practitioner: a good way to refine the technique. Afterall we can't fit strain gauges to the spines of our patients and clients.

Static stretching

Stretching is a common sight, both on the rehabilitation ward and on the sports field. Stretching a muscle is, generally, achieved by placing the muscle in its longest position, moving the relative attachments as far apart as possible. Achieving this position may require a little thought for muscles that extend over more than one joint, e.g. the hamstrings and calf muscles (see Fig. 10.4), but in general it's a pretty simple technique. But you could still make mistakes.

There are basic questions to be addressed when stretching, for example: how long should the stretch be held for? How many stretches a day are necessary? And should the tissue be warmed up before, during or after stretching? Insight to these questions comes from recalling our discussions on the viscoelastic nature of connective tissue. As you will remember, when the stretch is applied the tissues will deform (lengthen) and reform immediately (that's the elastic bit), but they will also allow

themselves to flow if the stress is maintained (that's the viscous bit). So if you want the stretch to last longer than the duration of the stretch itself then you must hold it for a period of time. Research suggests that a stretch should be held for at least 15 s to be effective; this amount of time is necessary for the tissue to creep. You will be glad to hear, however, that holding a stretch for more than 30 s is not any more effective.

It also appears from research that one stretch a day is sufficient to **maintain** flexibility although more frequent stretches may be required if an **increase** is desired. Finally, having your tissues warmed up makes the stretch more effective because they are less resistant to flow (i.e. less viscous), and it seems that being warm **during** the stretch is the critical thing.

Recalling our discussions in Chapter 7, we know that the stretched connective tissue returns to its original size and properties within an hour or two. Although this duration of increased flexibility varies across individuals, the point is that it is a short-lived improvement in muscle length. So why do it?

The three most widely held reasons for stretching are:

1. Improved joint mobility and therefore function;

2. Reduced risk of injury during participation in a sport or physical activity; and

3. Improved performance in a sport or physical activity.

While the first reason is perfectly valid (although more long-lasting solutions are sometimes required—see the section on orthoses, p. 129) the last two reasons have recently come under scrutiny. Stretching is a well-established part of the preparation for a physical activity such as a game of football; however, very little evidence exists to support its claim of either improving performance or reducing risk of injury. I will leave you with one thought on this subject, because it's good to be a little sceptical.

If you stretch a muscle/tendon you will have temporarily altered its stiffness. This improved flexibility may be a good thing for activities like gymnastics; however, reducing a tendon's stiffness will affect its ability to transfer force efficiently. The impact of this on sports performance is not entirely clear but it is certainly something to think about.

Respiratory techniques

Therapists don't just use force on the musculoskeletal system; those working with patients incapacitated with a respiratory condition also use force. The forced expiratory technique (FET), or simply called huffing for reasons soon to become obvious, is a technique employed by respiratory physiotherapists and nurses to help individuals get rid of excessive or thick mucus lining their airways which might be affecting their breathing. Basically the technique consists of one or two 'huffs' (see Practical Activity 10.3) interspersed between controlled breathing. The purpose is to generate high velocity in the air leaving your lungs. But why would you want to do that if you were trying to get rid of mucus? Two reasons:

1. Higher air speed creates more turbulent air flow and greater shear forces which could dislodge bits of mucus. It's like a fast-flowing wild river that can take bits of the river bank with it, bit of tree, mud, etc.

2. As well as dislodging bits of mucus the shear forces alter the viscosity of the mucus lining

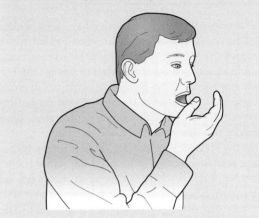

Figure 10.5 • The forced expiratory technique (FET).

the sides of the air tracts. This is gained through friction between the air and mucus which warms it up, like the way you warm up your hands by rubbing them together. The increased temperature reduces the viscosity of the mucus (makes it runnier), making it easier to cough up.

A simple analogy would be cleaning out a blocked drain pipe by pushing fast-flowing water through it. When you think about this, that is what you do when you cough, fast air flow, the FET is a refined version that avoids the trauma of harsh repetitive coughing.

CD-ROM activity 10.2

There are other respiratory techniques with a mechanical basis. Take the percussion technique for example. Although not as commonly used now, percussion is used by respiratory physiotherapists and nurses to help move secretions (mucus) that may have built up excessively on the wall of the airway, a symptom of a chest infection for example and one that reduces the functional capacity of the lung. So how does the percussion help?

In the percussion technique the therapist 'claps' the chest wall with a cupped hand and in so doing creates a sound wave (due to the compression of air against the chest wall) which is transmitted through the lung tissue to literally shake the mucus.

Again the effect may not simply be to dislodge the mucus but also to alter its viscosity.

Hydrotherapy

The therapeutic benefits of water have been widely used for thousands of years. In rehabilitation water provides a versatile medium suitable for a broad range of individuals, from older patients to young athletes. Buoyancy and drag can be used to construct exercise programmes that start with assisting and supporting movement and end with strenuous resistance. Let's consider the biomechanics of one technique.

In the Halliwick approach to hydrotherapy turbulence is used extensively to assist the patient. One example of this is where the therapist stands behind the patient who is lying on their back in the water, perhaps supported by floats (see Fig. 10.6). The therapist then begins to walk backwards, while providing some support to the patient's head (always re-assuring). The water between the therapist and patient becomes turbulent with a resulting drop in pressure (Bernoulli's principle—see Chapter 8), which pulls the patient towards the therapist (try Practical Activity 10.4 if you don't believe me).

Practical Activity Box 10.4

You can try this simple exercise in your bath. Put your rubber duck/toy boat in a bit of calm water (and free of bubbles), put your hand in the water a couple of centimetres in front of the duck and pull your hand through the water towards you. Do it slowly, and then do it quickly. Did the duck move? If not then try keeping your hand closer to the duck while you are moving. You are applying Bernoulli's principle to move the duck, creating fast-flowing turbulent water which has a lower pressure; this pressure difference causes a pulling force on the duck.

The purpose of this technique is to develop confidence and balance in the water, so the patient is moving through the water without much help from the therapist. They may then begin to contribute more to the movement by moving their hands and feet. It provides a really good starting point, and hey if it's good enough for ducklings then it should be good enough for us.

There are many other ways that a therapist can use water to facilitate or resist movement using buoyancy and drag in particular. Have a think about how you might, for example, resist shoulder abduction using buoyancy and drag (suggestions are in Appendix 10).

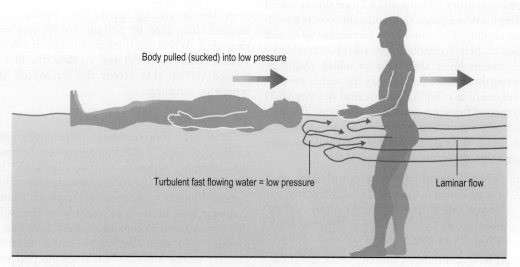

Body pulled (sucked) into low pressure

Turbulent fast flowing water = low pressure

Laminar flow

Figure 10.6 • Using Bernoulli's principle to assist swimming.

Orthoses

The Latin word *ortho* means straighten or correct. So, we have *ortho*dontistry, which is about straightening your teeth; *ortho*paedics, which is about straightening children—although this is the literal translation it generally means to straighten bones; it's just that children were the ones that traditionally had their bones straightened!

Orthoses are devices that correct or support parts of the musculoskeletal system. So this might be an insole in your shoe to prevent the arch in your foot from dropping too much when you are standing and walking or it could be a wrist support that limits the amount of flexion. They are made of different materials depending on their function. For example, a very flexible elastic insole, while providing some pressure relief, is unlikely to prevent the medial arch collapsing; this needs a certain amount of stiffness. Let's look at the biomechanics of one orthosis, the medial heel wedge which is mainly used by podiatrists to correct the position of the calcaneum (heel bone) during upright activities. As the name suggests this is a wedge of relatively stiff material lodged under the medial side of the calcaneum so that it tilts the calcaneum in a clockwise direction.

It should be noted that the magnitude of the forces acting on the foot when walking and running are likely to be too large for an external orthosis (i.e. one not fixed directly to the bones) such as the medial heel wedge to completely control foot posture. Rather than controlling the force an orthotic insole is regarded as a training device: to give the body a closer to normal sensation of where the force should be felt and which muscles should be working (and which shouldn't).

In Figure 10.7 you can see the position of the calcaneum. In normal circumstances the calcaneum

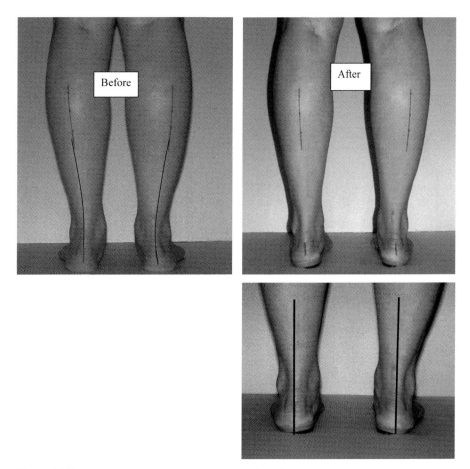

Figure 10.7 • Use of medial heel wedges to rotate the calcaneum.

should be, more or less, straight. In the figure it is clear that the calcaneum is rotated medially (also called abduction or valgus). Now, because the calcaneum is linked to the rest of the lower limb this rotation causes a domino effect throughout. You should be able to see this further up the leg in Figure 10.7.

You can feel this (albeit in reverse) for yourself. Take your shoes off and stand up. Now twist one whole leg in a little (left or right side, it doesn't matter) while keeping your weight on it. You should see (you may need a friend to help here) and feel that the calcaneum rotates and that your arch lowers to the ground. There you have it, a demonstration that the whole lower limb is linked up, if you didn't know already.

Obviously you did that for demonstration purposes but if you had to walk with a valgus calcaneum and flattened arch you would soon feel uncomfortable (in your whole lower limb). The purpose of the medial heel wedge is therefore to untwist (de-rotate) the calcaneum so that it sits more upright when standing (just the same as putting a couple of folded beer mats under the leg of a sloping table so that the drinks don't spill). Figure 10.7 shows this clearly and also the effect this de-rotation has higher up the limb.

Dynamic wrist splints

If it's good enough for the feet it's good enough for the hands. Of course splints are also used to apply and modify forces acting over the wrist and hand.

A good example of this is the dynamic wrist splints widely used, although not exclusively, by occupational therapists. These are essentially moulded plastic sleeves that wrap around the wrist and hand (see Fig. 10.8) sometimes with wires that create additional forces (Fig. 10.9). Their purpose, typically, is to apply tensile stress to shortened tissue. Because they are worn for prolonged periods they work on the viscoelastic properties of connective tissue, i.e. stress applied over time to give the tissue an opportunity to flow (see Chapter 7). Orthodontists use a similar approach when they fix braces to teeth; low load and prolonged duration mean the tissue won't be damaged and any changes in the length (or position in the case of teeth) are more likely to be permanent.

The makeup of the dynamic splint is quite interesting from a biomechanical perspective. First the plastic sleeve (Fig. 10.8) is 'thermodynamic'. This means that when it is heated it becomes very compliant (in exactly the same way that your own tissues are more flexible when warmer, just more so with the plastic) and, on cooling, will become stiff again (this, believe it or not, may also happen to our tissues but the research is still not conclusive). This allows the therapist to mould the sleeve carefully around wrist/hand. If you are going to apply force to a body part (even low loads over long periods) it is important to make sure the force is evenly spread; otherwise, there is a risk that some parts will experience higher pressure with resulting damage to the skin. A tight-fitting sleeve is also important to avoid the splint moving up and down which creates shear stress on the skin. Prolonged

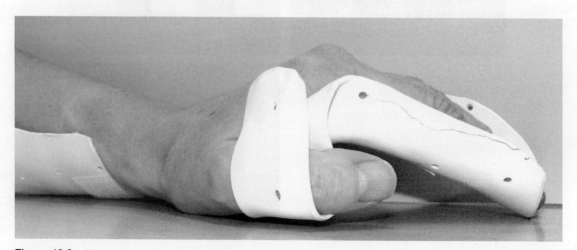

Figure 10.8 • Wrist splint moulded to hand to help maintain functional position of wrist.

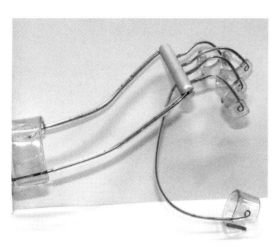

Figure 10.9 • The use of wires to generate additional stress along specific directions.

applications of shear stress are likely to result in skin damage—just like the blisters caused by your feet sliding up and down in shoes that are way too big.

The next part of the dynamic splint is the wires (see Fig. 10.9) which apply a force in a specific direction. The wires can be tightened a certain amount every time they see the therapist so that the tensile stress is maintained. Don't want any slacking off. If you recall Chapter 7, this was called tissue creep.

What you have learned from this

We have looked at a number of techniques used by health and sports professionals and examined the underpinning biomechanics. We found that the angle of application of a spinal mobilization would create rotation and some superficial soft tissue sliding rather than vertical displacement. The effectiveness of stretching was explained using its viscoelastic properties and some doubt introduced as to the use of stretching to improve sport performance (well, not in all sports anyway). We found that the respiratory technique 'huffing' used shear force and turbulence to dislodge mucus as well as make it less viscous. We also looked at the use of orthotics in sport and rehabilitation and found that they are used widely and successfully to *straighten* body parts, although the main benefits were re-training muscle activity rather than realigning bones.

The intention of this chapter, and in many ways the whole book, has been to give you greater insight into the biomechanics involved in your practice as a health or sports professional. The movement examples early in the book and example of techniques in this chapter are just that: examples. It is up to you now to apply these principles to other aspects of your practice. You have the knowledge.

Appendices

Appendix 1

Answers and explanations

The circled words in the following are vectors:

Speed   Depth   Circumference   (Displacement)

Length   (Force)   Luminosity   Distance

Mass   Heat   (Velocity)   (Acceleration)

Wind   Snowfall   Weight   Time

What about force **D** (40 N)?

Force **D** vector has a length of 4.76 cm, therefore a magnitude of 47.6 N. It is applied downwards at an angle of 37° to the horizontal (X) or 53° to the vertical (Y).

The answer to Practical Activity 1.3 is hand position D, since this provides the furthest distance from the knee joint, larger moment arm.

Appendix 2

- The lying down position would be easiest because the CoM is positioned directly above the joint centre. If you drew a vertical line down from the CoM it would pass through the joint. Just like a child sitting in the middle of a seesaw this produces compression but not a turning force (moment).
- If you want to gradually increase resistance from the lying down position, you could simply move the limb a little out of position, 80° rather than 90°. This would create small moments that the muscles have to resist. Why not try it for yourself: lie on your side and lift your arm directly up so that your fingers point to the ceiling. Feel how much muscle work is required and then move it a little closer to your body. Can you feel the moderate difference this makes?
- The order of difficulty for hip abduction, with the most difficult first, would be:

  1. Lying on 'good' side and lifting operated leg directly up into abduction.

  2. Lying on 'good' side with knee bent and moving leg directly up into abduction.

  3. Standing and moving operated leg out into abduction.

  4. Lying on back moving operated leg out into abduction (out to side).

- In Figure 2.12 the forward location of the CoM on the neck will create a flexor moment (the force is trying to bring the head down, chin down onto the chest). So to avoid this there must be an extensor moment created by activity in the neck extensors. The further forward the head is, the greater the

flexor moment induced by gravity, the greater the counteracting extensor moment. Increased muscle activity can result in compression of joints as well as discomfort within the muscles, particularly if they are asked to hold this position for prolonged periods. The solution is simple: educate the individual to hold their head in a more retracted position (head back) so that its CoM is placed closer to the neck joints.

- Can you think of any other situations when a wheelchair may become unstable?
- What would happen when moving down a slope?

Answer:

Moving down a slope will shift your CoG forwards so that it is closer to the forward limit of your BoS. There is a small risk that you could become unstable; however, leaning back into the chair is likely to be all that is required to ensure the CoG is maintained within the BoS. Leaning forwards is not advisable.

- What about hanging a rucksack on the handles at the back?

Answer:

Hanging a bag onto the back of your wheelchair shifts the CoM backwards. This means you are more prone to backward instability, e.g. when going up a slope or a pavement kerb.

- Or how about if the occupant becomes a lower-limb amputee?

Answer:

The loss of a lower limb means there is less mass located forwards, a topsy-turvy way of saying your CoM will move backwards, bringing it closer to the limit of the BoS at the back. This of course presents a greater possibility of destabilizing backwards. To combat this, wheelchairs for amputees are designed with their wheels positioned further back to extend the BoS backwards.

- Some tight rope artists hold a pole which is bent downwards. What do you think is the advantage of this?

Answer:

The reason for a pole that bends downwards is that as well as improving lateral stability it also lowers the CoM, making you more stable.

Appendix 3

- The correct force combination for the car push (Fig. 3.5) would be F4 and F5, adding the forces in both these combinations would produce the same force vector as Barry (F1).
- To stop the patella moving more towards one side than the other we need to make sure the resultant is straight. Because we can't alter the direction of the muscle (we would need the help of an orthopaedic surgeon for that) we can only achieve this by increasing the size of the vastus

medialis vector (by strengthening). We could try to reduce the size of vastus lateralis (weaken it) but this would mean resting the muscle which would also weaken vastus medialis. So we need specific exercises for vastus medialis, which is just what physiotherapists and sports therapists do.
- Simultaneous activation of the three parts of deltoid would result in a combined force similar to the figure below:

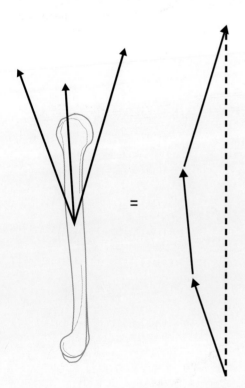

Appendix 4

• By bending the leg as it swings, the moment of inertia of the leg is reduced (therefore easier to swing) but it also helps in clearing the ground, an important factor in avoiding a trip fall.

Transfer of momentum from horizontal to vertical during the sit-to-stand movement

The momentum of the trunk, which is mainly horizontal, is transferred to the lower limbs through the action of the hip extensors (gluteus maximus and hamstrings). As the trunk flexes forwards these muscles are more and more wound up, like springs. They do what any spring would do when it is pulled at one end: they pull on the other end, which means extending (straightening) the thigh, which helps to lift your body up. Clearly this transfer is not sufficient to accomplish the vertical movement, so you also need input from the knee extensors (quadriceps) as well as active shortening of gluteus maximus and the hamstrings. Nonetheless this is a highly efficient use of the body's momentum. Energy and efficiency will be explored more in Chapter 9.

Appendix 5

Question 2

A hoist is used to lift a disabled customer weighing 105 kg into a swimming pool. How much work does the hoist perform when lifting the man 1.7 m up?

Answer:

Magnitude of force = mass (105 kg) × acceleration (9.81) = 1030 N.

The work done is 1030 N × 1.7 (displacement) = 10,104.3 J.

Question 3

An angler catches a fish. The fish pulls hard on the end of the line and the angler begins to turn his reel (the pulley mechanism at the end of the rod) to bring the fish into shore. He pulls on the handle with 90 N; the handle is 0.064 m from the centre of the reel. The circumference of the reel is 40 cm. The man turns the reel three times to lift the fish. How much work does he perform?

Answer

Displacement	= 3 × 0.4 (circumference)	= 1.2 m
Rotational force	= 90 × 0.064 = 5.76 Nm	
Work done	= 18.75 rad (526°) × 5.76	
	= 108 J of work	

Question 4

A man is holding a 2-kg tin of chopped tomatoes in his hand. The combined mass of the tomatoes and his forearm is 6 kg, which produces a force of 6 × 9.81 = 58.9 N. This force is located approximately 40 cm from the elbow. The combination of force and distance from joint creates an extension moment (rotational force trying to straighten the elbow) 58.9 N × 0.4 = 23.5 Nm. The elbow flexors (muscles that bend the elbow) apply their opposing rotational force (flexor moment) at a closer distance, i.e. 5 cm.

To hold the tomatoes steady the elbow flexors must produce a force of at least 23.5 Nm; otherwise, the arm will fall down (a bit like the seesaw in CD-ROM activity 1.3).

23.5 Nm = 0.05 × ?

Therefore

23.5/0.05 = 470 N!

Categories of levers

1. Modern cranes are generally type 3 levers: there are many types of crane in existence but in essence they all work on the same principle of levers providing mechanical advantage so it is easier to lift an object.

2. Scissors are an example of a type 1 lever: the effort (you pressing) is on one side of the pivot and the load (paper, etc.) is on the other; scissors can also be described as a double lever since there are two of them working together.

3. A bottle opener is an example of a type 2 lever: your effort is at one end, the pivot point is at the other and the load/resistance is between the two.

4. The drawbridge of a castle is a type 2 lever: the load (mass of the bridge) is placed between the pivot and the effort (where the chain is attached).

Practical activity 5.1

The triceps are actually working as a type 1 lever, effort (attachment of triceps) is behind the joint and the load (mass of arm) is in front.

Answers to practical problems on force and human movement

Inserting a sock under your heel shifted the centre of pressure forwards. The centre of pressure can be considered to be the point of application of the ground reaction force (GRF). By moving this forwards it will alter the moments acting about the lower limb joints. When standing normally (i.e. no sock under your heel) the GRF lies slightly (4 or 5 cm) in front of the ankle (Figs. 2.7 and 2.13), causing a small dorsiflexing moment (i.e. your ankle feels like it wants to bend), which is counterbalanced (otherwise you would fall forward!) by a plantarflexing moment (see Fig. 1.12) provided by the muscles behind your ankle (also known as the plantarflexors). Moving the centre of pressure forwards increases the size of this dorsiflexing moment, which, unless you don't want to fall forwards, means much more activity in the plantarflexors, which you may feel after a while.

Walking backwards means the forefoot strikes the ground first (as opposed to the heel). Normally the heel strike creates a plantarflexing moment because it is located behind the ankle (so there is corresponding activity of the dorsiflexors). Hitting the ground with your forefoot, however, means this will be reversed, so you will get a dorsiflexing moment and consequently (like the last question) more activity in the plantarflexors. Because the foot is being lowered when you hit the ground the muscles perform negative work; they are still active to control the moment but are allowing the joint to move (in a controlled manner) in the opposite direction.

Bending forwards (stooping) when you are standing alters many things which you can easily feel. In very basic terms you have moved your CoM forwards. If you think about your stability (Practical Activity 2.7) this may make you unstable, but really you would have to bend forward a lot to make you topple forwards because a lot of your base of support (feet) is in front of you. Why not try it for yourself? Stand up and see how far forwards you need to bend before you begin to feel like you are falling forwards. The problem with stability and this posture comes when you start to walk.

During gait, at the point of impact with the ground, the body decelerates (change in momentum); this deceleration starts at the foot and moves up the body (like a wave) so that the upper body continues to move forwards a little after the foot has stopped. This doesn't last long and the body quickly reverts to the efficient upside-down pendular motion with the body rotating forwards over a fixed foot, as discussed in Chapter 9. The problem comes when you have already moved the CoM forwards (when you are in a stooped posture); this continued motion of the body after initial contact risks a forwards instability (you might fall forwards) with the CoM now much closer to the front limit of the base of support. Again why not try this? Bend forwards again, at your hip, and walk. You may experience a sensation of toppling forwards when your foot lands. This might reveal itself in an increased urgency to take the next step.

Now some individuals are forced into this flexed/stooped posture because of a spinal condition; however, puzzlingly it seems that some people deliberately adopt this posture. This is a strategy not borne from vanity or efficiency but rather a specific impairment of the lower limbs. If you lose enough strength in your quadriceps muscle (through injury or disease) it means the body is unable to resist the large flexing moment created by the GRF vector projecting behind the knee joint. By moving the CoM forwards the GRF is less angled so it comes closer to the knee joint, creating a smaller moment, so less is required from the knee extensors (quadriceps). Why not try it out and see what you think? A similar change in knee moments could be achieved by hitting the ground with your forefoot first but I will leave you to work out how that works. Remember trying things out helps a lot.

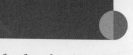 CD-ROM activity 5.7

Trying to stand up with your legs further forward than normal (because of a friendly dog) will feel like much harder work than normal, simply because you are moving your body a greater distance forwards (work is force × distance). To make this bigger jump you need to generate larger moments about your lower limb joints as well as more contribution from your upper body (throwing arms forward, etc.). Because of the more forward location of the ground reaction force the moment at your knee may be extensor (GRF orientated in front of your knee), whereas normally it would be flexor.

We have all come across the slippery floor situation so we all know that to avoid slipping we do two things, usually. We slow down and we take smaller steps. These two, not necessarily related, strategies reduce the risk of falling by altering the size and direction of force applied by your body to the ground. By slowing down, the change in momentum at initial contact (and pre-swing—see CD-ROM activity 5.6 for reminder of gait phases) is much reduced so the force magnitude is reduced. By taking smaller steps the angle of the GRF is more vertical (like you are stamping your legs straight down); therefore the horizontal component (which will cause your slip) will be reduced. Reduced magnitude and reduced angle of the GRF means less chance of slipping.

Appendix 6

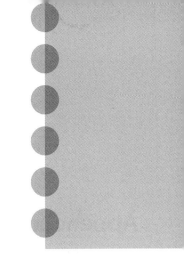

(A) The foot while jogging

- What kind of stress does the anteroposterior horizontal component cause at the metatarsal heads?
  - ○ Bending
  - ○ Torsional
  - ○ Shear*
  - ○ Compressive
- What kind of stress does the vertical component cause at the metatarsal heads?
  - ○ Bending
  - ○ Torsional
  - ○ Shear
  - ○ Compressive*
- What could happen with repetitive stress application?

Repetitive compressions can lead to callus (thickened skin) formation. This is the body's response to this kind of stress. Areas of high compressive stress can lead to corns forming.

Repetitive applications of the shear stress can lead to the skin breaking down with inflamed skin and possibly blisters.

(B) A blow to back of knee

Imagine you are attending a game of soccer. You see a particularly bad tackle with one player kicking the back of the knee of another player causing the tibia to slide forwards.

- What type of stress is experienced by the articular surface from the movement of the tibia?

Shear stress

- What type of stress does the anterior cruciate experience? The anterior cruciate is a strong ligament orientated to prevent the tibia sliding forward.

Tensile stress

- What do you think might happen to the anterior cruciate with this kind of stress?

Tearing of the ligament, usually at its weakest point, which is where it attaches to the bone.

Appendix 7

Creep is an effective way of gaining a lot of elongation from a tissue; however, it makes the tissue less stiff. If this decrease in stiffness occurred at the tendons then this would effect its ability to transfer the force of the muscle to turning the bone, which may have a detrimental effect on performance of a sport or even put the tissue at risk of injury because, for a short period (60–90 minutes) it is not as strong as it was. This suggests a small number of repetitions should be used and that these should not be done before engagement in an activity which involves large forces, such as participation in a sport.

Dynamic stretching

Repetitive or cyclical stretching used to be called dynamic or ballistic stretching and was discouraged due to the risk of injury. However, it has been re-introduced for particular sports and activities where the tissues experience highly repetitive stretching, e.g. triple jump, volleyball and basketball. In these sports dynamic stretching is now well practised because it trains the elastic recoil characteristics of the muscles involved in repetitive stretching, e.g. gastrocnemius.

Appendix 8

What are cyclists trying to achive with the following?

1. Smooth skin-hugging clothes.
   Reduce friction (well, that's what they say).
2. Bikes smoothed with the joints in the frame rounded.
   Reduce friction.
3. Low riding position, back flat and crouched over the handle bars.
   Reduce form drag (there may also be an improved ability to generate more powerful leg extension).
4. A back wheel that is filled in with a disk.
   Reduce form drag. Quite a lot of turbulence is created by the revolving spokes so disc wheels can reduce this (not always a good idea, particularly if cycling with a side wind).
5. Helmets shaped like a teardrop at the back.
   Reduce form drag (as well as making you look like an extra from a science fiction movie).
6. Riders cycling very closely behind each other.
   Take advantage of negative pressure (this can reduce the effort of cycling by as much as 40%).
7. Shaved legs.
   Reduce friction (although any reduction is minimal).

Appendix 10

Shoulder adduction (bringing your arm to your side) could be resisted firstly with drag. Lying on your back (using appropriate floats) with your arm lying out to the side move it slowly back to your side. The resistance to your movement came from (a) the mass of the water you are pushing out the way and (b) drag, mainly from friction. Now do the same movement faster. This will be harder because of an increase in drag (mass of displaced water will be the same) from the turbulent flow created by the faster movement.

There is, of course, a limit to how much you can use drag; afterall you can only go so fast. So to increase the resistance further you could use buoyancy. From a standing position, with arm out to the side (so the arm is lying on top of the water) pull your arm down to your side. This movement is resisted by buoyancy. To progress the resistance you can make the arm bigger (so more water is displaced) and make the arm lighter (relative density is decreased). This is accomplished nicely with an inflatable arm band. The more air in the arm band, the greater the resistance from buoyancy during the adduction movement.

Index

NB: Page numbers in **bold** refer to boxes, figures and tables